BEDTIME STORIES FOR ADULTS

RELAXING SLEEP STORIES TO CALM YOUR MIND AND FALL IN A RESTFUL DEEP SLEEP. OVERCOME INSOMNIA, OVERTHINKING, AND POWERFUL GUIDED MEDITATIONS TO DEFEAT ANXIETY AND DAILY STRESS

GWENDA K. WOOD

CONTENTS

INTRODUCTION

Regardless of whether a story is amusing, dismal, unnerving or unusual, they give kids something to think about. At the point when we do it at sleep time, we likewise give our youngsters the solid message that we care for them. Right now of 'separation' (saying 'goodnight') we are stating that we are 'appended' (we're there for them).

Michael Rosen's We're Going on a Bear Hunt

Obviously, another perspective pretty much this is it's everything darned great fun. Probably the best occasions you'll ever have – regardless of whether that is as a parent, grandparent, more seasoned kin or parent – is sharing a story at sleep time. Also, from the kid's perspective, as that kid grows up, it'll be one of the most wonderful recollections you'll ever have of those individuals who set aside the effort to impart stories to you.

What are you most loved sleep time stories? Are there any that you recollect from your adolescence or that your kids love to hear? Assuming this is the case, at that point don't hesitate to tell us in the remarks.

Much like some tea, there's almost no a decent book can't explain - a work situation, a culinary groove and even, (most eminently for somebody like me, who used to battle to get enough shut-eye), an awful night's rest. Making my Kindle a fundamental piece of my pre-rest routine assumed a significant job in making something happen, be that as it may, changing from printed copy to sound could help improve the nature of my sleep considerably more.

A key explanation? It's more in line with how the body normally turns off. "As we rest, our hearing sense is one of the last things to close down," clarifies Hope Bastine, inhabitant clinician for rest innovation brand, Simba. "It's likewise the principal sense to return the morning – which is the reason hearing the winged creatures twittering is frequently what carry your brain to awareness. Utilizing sound at night constantly serves to efficiently close down the remainder of the faculties and better readies the brain and body for that natural rest state."

Swapping paper for a couple of earphones additionally gives a truly necessary pocket of idealism if your way of life's a little workstation overwhelming right now. "Our screen-age society implies our eyes are progressively exhausted around evening time," remarks Hope. So if tech's negatively affecting your eyes, perusing with your ears could give an all the more loosening up approach to pacify your internal savant.

CHAPTER 1

Soupy

Sleep is an odd concept when Adam started think about it. It's something that all humans and animals have to do to keep their energy and sanity up, and it seems like it would be simple as closing your eyes and letting yourself drift to the world beyond our consciousness. Just slowly droop those eyes, let your mind wander a bit, and then you seamlessly enter the world of sleep.

However, that rarely happened for Adam. After a day at the job, he'd get himself comfortable. Take off his work clothes and throw them into some part of the house designated to be the hamper this time. Then, he'd pour himself a nice cup of soupy tea. Herbal tea designed to calm the mind and allow relaxation.

Adam plopped the tea bag into the kettle and watched everything heat up, the lukewarm tap water transforming into a soupy feast of herbal goodness. Sometimes, he'd sprinkle a bit of stevia in there for the sweetness, but other times, he tended to enjoy his tea as it was.

The sound of tea pouring was a welcome one, and as his cup with a realistic cat face contained it, he'd curl up in his couch and watch some of his favorite shows. Sometimes, he'd watch a nature documentary. Ah, to be like an animal and rely only on instinct on not this hybrid that humans are. Ah, to be a fish and never have to worry about what the land animals were up to. Ah, to be a creature who could easily get sleep.

Other times, he may watch a more complex show. Something with intricate character arcs that would weave around like a child who didn't know how to tie his shoes, going in all sorts of directions. If the show was good, it may have kept Adam up a little longer, but if it was a boring little bottle episode, then he'd feel the weight on his eyes.

Adam wasn't picky. He'd watch reality shows that rotted your brain from within, he'd watch slice of life anime in a language he possibly couldn't learn. He'd watch everything the TV would throw at him, all while sipping some tea.

Sometimes, he'd look around for something to watch, and nothing would please his palate. Imagine if you will, going to a buffet, and yet all the food around you is as appealing as walking around the beach wearing a parka. In a case like that, he may have switched to some music. Nothing to rock out with, but instead ambient beats or calm classical music.

As he sipped his tea, the music helped him focus, and he would review his day. Being a white-collar working man, he didn't have too much to review. Sometimes, there may have been a funny incident at the office, such as the time when Marlee brought a bunch of donuts, only for the donuts to have been days old due to Marlee always forgetting to bring them.

Other times, his mind may wonder into a little more something with meat in it. As the notes of the classical music wrapped around his brain, he looked back in his thirtysomething odd years and wondered if things could be better. He was a single man, living in an apartment, all with his cat, Purrito. Speak of the devil.

Purrito, at this point, would hop on his lap. Purrito was a white cat with specks of brown, sort of resembling a burrito if you will. If Adam forgot to feed Purrito, the cat would come up next to him, conveniently as he was about to relax, and let out her cries. At first, Adam may have meowed back, but he realized that he couldn't feed Purrito with his meows.

Instead, Adam stood up and went to the cupboard. There, he located the cat food. Meow Crisp, a crunchy cat concoction. He scooped up a cup, hearing the rattling of the food in the bag, and then he poured it into Purrito's polka dotted bowl. The sound of it pouring brought a sort of warmth to Adam, and he smiled as Purrito munched on her meal.

After that detour, he'd retreat to his couch, where he would once again reminisce. Perhaps he should follow his dreams, as the cliché went. While he was still a relatively young man, those years were right behind him. Like relaxing on a beach, letting the waves kiss your feet, only to realize that the big tidal wave was coming.

Adam let out a yawn. Every night, he was a little too tired to think about what he wanted to do. He wanted to provide a community service or do something, but what? Anything sounded better than his generic office job.

Another yawn. This time, right as he took a sip of the soupy tea. It felt like he was breathing fire, as the tea had a slight heat to it. The time was almost here. Adam would soon attempt to go to sleep, and maybe he could get it right the first time.

Adam let out another yawn, and another. At this point, Purrito was no longer hungry, and she walked up to Adam. Adam patted her back, and felt the vibration emanating from it. Cat purrs were the ultimate drug you could never get tired of. Laying your hand on your happy little cat, you could just feel the purrs leaving the cat's body and going into yours, vibrating their way to your heart, giving it a warm sensation. He smiled, and then yawned again. Downing his tea, he yawned once more.

Twas time. Adam walked to the bathroom and brushed his teeth. The rhythmic brushing was a song that indicated that it was time to go to bed. Ah. Minty freshness spread throughout his mouth, thc foaming toothpaste being a chunky soup in its own regard. After performing the toothbrush ritual, Adam went to his bed. A full-sized bed, it wasn't the biggest thing, but it was enough to contain Adam and had some softness to it, so he was satisfied. He turned on his lamp, crawled into bed, and whipped out a book.

Every book he had was about something mundane, like finances, or a generic self-help book. He figured he'd give his eyes a bit of relaxation from the screen and instead focus on the inked pages of a book. Books could be exciting, taking you to a magical world of make-believe, but they could also be boring, like a self-help book telling you over and over again that you could do it. In this case, it was the latter.

Soon, the waves of tiredness hit Adam. It was like being on a dock on a foggy, soupy day, and in the distance, he could hear the sounds of the foghorn telling you that his ship had arrived. He'd soon step on it, and then go into the unknown that was the world of dreams. He turned on his fan, and as the white noise filled the room, he shut off his lamp, and the darkness filled the room. Ah. The room was the perfect temperature, balancing out the cool air with the warm blankets. Adam got on his side. He had a good feeling about tonight. He closed his eyes.

Flip. Flip. Flip.

Flipping the pillow, flipping himself around, flipping off the forces responsible for human sleep. Everything was about flipping. While he was initially tired, and he thought it would be a sure journey to dream world, he realized that his ship hadn't arrived yet. In fact, he had some energy. It was that burst of energy that popped out of a sea of tiredness, like someone struggling to get out of quicksand, but it was enough to keep him awake.

Adam studied about insomnia and realized that he had to get up and do something. When you sleep, the last thing you want is to stay in bed, as your brain likes to associate restlessness with your bed. Human brains were odd that way, he supposed. He stood up and followed his trail of nightlights to the bathroom, them guiding him like a starry sky. He flipped on the lights, the lights emitting a dull little glow, perfect for a quiet bathroom setting.

He soon poured the bathwater. Adam was a morning shower type of person, but when insomnia bit him, he bit back with a bath. The soupy, hot water began filling the tub, the water's flowing trading off with another yawn from Adam, but Adam knew that it probably wasn't time to go to bed just yet. He had to go to bed as soon as he knew he was ready. Whatever ready was.

The sound of water flowing into the bathtub was one that made Adam feel some kind of contentment. The water flowing washed away the neurons in his mind that collided over petty issues, such as that time he embarrassed himself in high school when he decided to wear clothes with their tags on them still. He knew as soon as he entered the soupy tub, it would be all better.

Soon, the tub was filled enough, and he even poured a little bit of foaming bath. The foam, radiating a smell of milk and honey, was like the icing on the cake, and soon Adam lied in it and collapsed in the soup. It was nice and toasty, yet not hot enough to feel like he was a part of someone's next meal. Adam propped himself up against the bathtub pillow and closed the curtain. As he did so, less light entered his domain. He was in the lair of the tub, where the soupy water would wash away his troubles.

He lied there, as the water sloshed around, and started thinking a bit about his day. As he did so, Purrito hopped on the side of the tub, let out a cute meow, dipped her paw in the bathtub, and licked from it with some grace. The sound of her scratchy tongue lapping at the water was another recipe in the sleepy cocktail that was his insomnia ritual. It felt so nice, and Adam sort of wished this would never end. But soon, tiredness hit him again.

He stayed a bit longer in there though. In the half-asleep world of insomnia, time was irrelevant. It could pass very fast as you were trying to go to bed or stop in moments like these. He let the soup of the tub grace his skin a little more, and his thoughts became a bit more jumbled. Instead of worrying, he was imagining himself on a beach, and on a mountain, or whatever guided imagery the podcast told him this week would help him sleep.

Darkness enveloped him, and he opened his eyes as he realized that the tub was not the best place to sleep. Using his foot, Adam pulled down the drain lever, and stayed in the tub, watching the soupy water around him lower, no longer kissing his skin with its warmth. Covered in water and a bit of foam, Adam went out of the tub, brushing his body with a towel. Soon, Adam yawned again, and went to bed.

He closed his eyes. Initially, there was a little more tossing and turning. There always was. Adam knew that sleep didn't come easy these days, and the only way to beat it was with acceptance. It sounded a bit like a cliché, but insomnia really was a tough cycle if you decided to fight against it. The only thing you could do was accept that sometimes, your body wants to fight against you. We are contradictory creatures after all, and our journey to get a full night's rest was just one of the many struggles of humans. It made sense for Adam, and Adam just imagined himself walking across a soupy swamp.

This swamp had all the contradictions lined up in a neat little row. One man sloshed through the swamp of wanting to go to sleep but can't sleep. Another woman paddled across the part of the swamp of having too much time, yet not having enough.

Instead of taking a dive in the soupy swamp, Adam proceeded to go somewhere else. He knew everyone had their swamp they were swimming in, unable to get out despite the outside being so much better. So instead, Adam kept walking. This swamp, as they said, went on for a long while. A long while. Many travelers would give up and wanted to take a dip in the swamps surrounding them. But Adam kept trotting through the marshlands, wondering where he was going. Could he find his way out?

As he continued to walk, one of his friends waved it him. It was Dave, swimming in the swamp of wanting to make time to hang out, but the bar was too tempting.

“The soup is fine,” Dave invited.

“No thanks,” Adam said. I have to keep going. With that, Adam went away, leaving Dave to do flips in the swamp.

He kept walking down the swamp, and at some point, nothing but swamp surrounded him. The marshlands had a clearing, a white light, right in front of him, but to get through it, he had to swim through the swamp. The soupy swamp of trying so hard yet trying not hard enough.

Adam dipped his toe in the swamp. It did have a creamy texture to it, but as he did so, temptation filled his body. He would stay in this swamp forever, would he not? There was no way out. He sat down. Maybe the swamp life wasn’t so bad after all. We all have our soup we have to swim in, and maybe his wasn’t so bad. He proceeded to roll into the swamp, when he heard a sound.

Reow!

He turned around. Purrito was behind him, but this time, Purrito was giant. She was the size of a noble steed. Adam walked next to Purrito and booped her on her giant pink nose, and vibrations emanated from this feline. Adam smiled, and he climbed aboard Purrito, using her fur as a way to hop on. Climb, climb, climb.

When he was on top, Adam pointed to the light at the end of the swamp. Purrito did not respond at first, but then Adam snapped his fingers. A laser pointer appeared his hands. He pointed it at the end, and Purrito wiggled her butt. Then, she took a mighty leap towards the light. As he soared high into the sky, Adam realized he had left the swamp, and now he was free from everything, free from-

His eyes opened just as Purrito pounced on his stomach. Just as she did, the alarm rang, and she ran off. Rubbing the sleepiness from his eyes, Adam had to chuckle. Another odd night of sleep, and he wouldn’t have it any other way, to be honest.

CHAPTER 2

Something Is Different

Hannah wakes up one morning and something is funny. Something feels different than usual. But what is it? Hannah looks around. Everything is in its place. The night light is on the bedside table and Bruno is sitting on the floor next to the bed.

Bruno is Hannah's favorite stuffed animal. A little white dog with a straw hat and dungarees. For a long time Bruno slept in bed. But Hannah is growing and so is not as much space in bed as before. In addition, Hannah is firmly convinced that Bruno has told her that he prefers to take care of her at night instead of sleeping. And that's a good thing - think Hannah!

Hannah slips off the bed, barefoot on the carpet. The carpet also feels as it always has. Funny! But no matter, Hannah thinks. She grabs Bruno under the arm and runs to mom and dad in the bedroom.

With a proper jump she jumps into the parents' bed and shouts, "Get up! I'm awake!". Hannah's mom and dad are still very sleepy. "Are you hungry honey?" Mum asks. Hannah thinks. "Hm, I think I could eat pancakes." Mum laughs: "We can not quite do it my darling. Today is kindergarten again. But tomorrow is the weekend. I'd like to make some pancakes for you. "

Hannah snaps her arms up: "Yes, weekend and pancakes." Then she jumps off the bed. "Come on Mom. We make breakfast fast and then kindergarten. Then it's really weekend! "

On the way to the kitchen Hannah tells her mom what happened today - that anything feels weird. Mom touches Hannah's forehead. "Hm. So - you do not have a fever. Take A. "Hannah opens her mouth wide and sticks out her tongue:" Ahhhhhhh. "But Mom shakes her head. "Everything's fine, too," she says.

As Hannah bites into the breakfast sandwich, she is startled. "Ow!" She calls. "What's up?" Mum asks. Hannah touches her finger in her mouth. "Hoa." She says with her finger in her mouth. Then she pulls out her finger. "There's a tooth wobbling!" She says indignantly.

Mama smiles: "Oh, you have a wiggle tooth. That explains a lot. Show me. "But Hannah quickly closes her mouth and shakes her head. Then she says, "No! I do not want to go to the dentist. "Mama strokes her cheek. "Darling, you do not have to go to the dentist with a wiggle."

Hannah makes big eyes. "Not?" She asks. "No!" Says Mom. "A jiggle falls out by itself. And when the time comes, we put it under your pillow at night. "" Ieeeee! "Interrupts Hannah's mom. "I'm not putting my tooth under my pillow."

Again, the mother smiles and says: "But only then can the tooth fairy get him. The next morning the tooth is gone and there is a coin there. "Hannah looks at Mum in disbelief. "Why is that?" She asks. "Because the tooth fairy does it," Mama answers.

Hannah does not quite understand that. "A fairy fetches my tooth and gives me money for it?" That makes Hannah think. "How much do I get for a tooth?" And immediately her finger disappears in her mouth again. "Uond waviel teeth hoeh ich then?"

"Enough to get rich," Mom jokes. But Hannah does not take that as a joke. "I knew it!" She calls and rubs her hands.

At kindergarten, Hannah eagerly talks about the Tooth Fairy. Jonas says tiredly: "Oh, about Zahnfee. This is definitely a mouse that steals the tooth. "But what does Jonas know? Jonas is stupid, thinks Hannah.

"Not at all!" Sandra intervened suddenly. "I've already put a tooth under my pillow and the next day there was money and the tooth was gone. So! "Then Jonas sticks out her tongue:" Bäääääh! "

Nevertheless, Hannah's sentence does not go out of her mind all day long. When Daddy picks up Hannah, she folds her arms and says, "I do not want a mouse to go under my pillow." Daddy looks at Hannah in amazement. "What mouse?" He asks. "Well, the tooth mouse." Hannah answers precociously. "Jonas says there is no tooth fairy. If I put my wiggle tooth under my pillow, then a mouse comes and fetches it. "

"Oh, Hannah," Dad says. "There is no tooth mouse! Do not listen to everything that's being told. "Hannah's stomach growls as loud as a bear. "Have not you eaten anything?" Dad asks in astonishment. Hannah turns away: "When I eat, my tooth falls out and then the mouse comes!"

Hannah's dad squats down and nudges Hannah. "The only mouse here is you," he whispers. "If your tooth is under the pillow, there comes a beautiful tiny little fairy. She is very happy about your tooth. And because you no longer need him, she buys him from you. That's all."

Hannah turns to her daddy: "And you are quite sure?" Hannah's father smiles and nudges her again: "Absolutely!" He says in a firm voice. "Alright! Then I want a huge dinner now. "Says Hannah and pulls her arms apart.

A few days later, it is actually time. Hannah's Wackelzahn finally falls out while eating. Hannah is really excited. She was never as fast at bed-making as she is today. When Mama says good night and begins to read a story, Hannah is fidgeting all the time. "What's going on?" Asks Hannah's mom. "I do not know exactly where to put my tooth down," she says restlessly, holding up her wobble tooth.

Hannah's mom takes the tooth and puts it under the pillow. "Well my sweatheart. Here he is exactly right. But now listen to the story and then sleep well. Because the fairy only comes when you sleep. "Hannah nods and listens to the story. "I can not sleep tonight," she thinks. But before she knows it, she has already fallen asleep.

The next morning she wakes up and slides barefoot on the floor. When she feels the carpet, she suddenly remembers the wobbly tooth. She quickly reaches for the pillow to check. The tooth is actually gone. She pulls the pillow off the bed and at the same moment she hears something falling on the carpet - a coin. She looks at the coin in amazement and whispers: "The tooth fairy was there." Then she grabs the money and runs happily to her parents. Again and again she calls, "They exist. Look, they really exist! "She runs straight into her daddy's arms. "Ui, with so much energy." Dad says as he takes Hannah up. Mom is making breakfast. "I said that," she laughs.

Hannah struggles with her legs. This is the sign for dad to let her down again. Once at the bottom, she stands straight up and holds the coin up. "I will show Jonas. He'll look around, "she says cheekily and everyone laughs heartily.

Then Hannah thinks for a moment and says: "Do you know what? I will always put all my wobbly teeth under my pillow. And when I'm rich, we all go ice cream! "Mom and Dad think the idea is great, and Hannah is proud to have lost her first shaky tooth - or rather, to have sold!

CHAPTER 3

Baggi's Unwanted Slide

Baggi loves to dig big holes. For that Baggi is still such a small excavator, he is already really fast. Once he grows up, he wants to be as big and strong a digger as his dad. The dredge huge pile of soil and debris in no time from one end of the construction site to another. The construction workers needed it for days. A strong excavator, like Baggis Papa, can do it in a few hours.

Baggi likes helping his dad with digging and so he has been to construction sites often. So often that he knows the environment like his own shovel. But that does not mean that things do not go wrong again and again.

Today, a house is to be built. For that the construction workers need a big hole in the earth. Said and done. Baggi gets going. Although he can dig really fast, he has to work hard to keep up with his daddy. Shovel by shovel, the hole grows larger quickly. Shovel after shovel but it is also fast deep. Baggi is so energetic and anxious to show his father what he is capable of, that he becomes overzealous.

He rolls faster and faster between the dug earth and the hole. It starts to drizzle. Baggis dad calls for a bad-weather break immediately - because safety first! But Baggi is at it right now and does not dream of stopping now.

But the wetter the earth gets, the slipperier it will be. Suddenly Baggi starts to skid. With momentum he rushes towards the hole. Even frightened by the unwanted slide and full of effort the little Baggi tries to slow down. But once you're in the slip, even the best brake will not help.

Baggi has an idea. He pushes his little shovel with all his strength into the ground. Now he is pulling a deep furrow and an ever-increasing pile of mud behind him. So the little Baggi tries to brake. And his plan seems to work out too, because he is getting bit by bit slower.

But unfortunately he came too late to this brilliant idea, because on the edge of the hole he is now on the loose and desperately trying to shift his weight forward so as not to slip into the huge hole.

Baggis slide was so fast that Baggis dad had not heard the fast-paced drama. Seeing Baggi on the tip, he rushes to his son's aid immediately. The wet ground does not make it easy for him. And so he comes to a tire length too late. Directly in front of him the small excavator slides straight into the hole. Behind him slips the wet earth, which he had accumulated during the slide.

Smudged and smudged with mud and earth, the little excavator now squats in the huge hole. As much as he tries to come out again, he finds no support. The wheels spin in the wet soil and he digs deeper into the earth. Even his strong dad can not reach him now.

"Just stay calm my boy. We'll get you out of there! "Shouts Baggis dad. Then he looks up and sees the construction workers standing on the other side of the hole. They are sprinkled with mud from top to bottom. Baggi had been so eager to get out of the hole that the mud had flown in a high arc to the construction workers. These now stand like drowned poodles on the edge and wipe the muddy ground from the face.

But on the job site, fortunately, one is a big family and not at all resentful. Because especially during construction can go something wrong. The important thing is that you help each other then.

The foreman taps the dirt from the radio. Then he immediately informs the crane driver: "Excavator in need!". The crane operator sees what is going on and swings the crane over the hole to free Baggi from his predicament.

Happy to have solid ground under the wheels, Baggi is relieved. But he is also embarrassed. For one thing, he should have listened to the security regulations and thus his dad. And on the other hand, everyone will surely make fun of him and tell funny stories about him.

But to Baggis astonishment no one makes fun of him. But on the contrary. Everyone is really worried about the little excavator and asks him if everything is alright and how it happened? Baggi tells the story from the beginning. After a while, he realizes that he is telling a funny story about himself. And that is really funny! The construction workers have a lot of fun listening to Baggis story. And since it is raining right now, no more work is done today anyway. But still laughed a lot and Baggi laughs heartily with! One bed free and one for three?

Today I tell you a story about a little girl named Lydia. Lydia is 4 years old and always nice and good. Mom and Dad are very proud that they have such a sweet child. Mum often even says "My Angel" to Lydia, because she is as good as an angel. But there is one thing that mom and dad do not find so divine. Lydia sleeps in her parents' bed every night.

How come? Surely you are asking yourself now. Does not she have her own bed? But she has. And even a very cuddly. With many stuffed animals and a lot of space for such a little girl as Lydia. But Lydia just does not want to sleep in her own bed. She finds it much more comfortable with mom and dad.

At the same time, Lydia does not know what it's like to sleep in her own bed. That was so long ago that she forgot.

Mom and dad love Lydia very much. But as big as mom and daddy's bed is, it's a little tight for three. Especially since Lydia gets bigger and bigger. When the dad turns around at night, he nudges Lydia. Then Lydia awakens briefly and turns around too. She bumps into her mom and the mom is awake and turns around. And when dad turns around again, the game starts again.

Sometimes Lydia twitches in her sleep. She then dreams something and begins to fidget with her arms and legs. Lydia herself does not notice. But depending on how she's lying, either mom or dad is lucky enough to get hit. Of course one wakes up on it. And if you do not sleep enough, you are not well rested in the morning.

If Lydia wants to play during the day, mom and dad are way too broken. You did not sleep much. And it was exhausting enough to do the work and the household.

Lydia thinks that's stupid. The solution would be so simple. She would only have to sleep in her own bed. Then mom and dad would have slept well and cheerful enough to play with Lydia.

Lydia used to sleep in her own bed when she was younger. There she liked to cuddle with her teddy. But Lydia does not remember that. At some point she got a new bed - because she got bigger. And she did not sleep once in the new bed.

If Mama Lydia had asked her if she would like to sleep in her own bed, then Lydia said, "No." Lydia said more. But today Mama said something for the first time that made Lydia think. "Your teddy is certainly very sad and misses you very doll."

Lydia did not even think that when she sleeps with Mom and Dad, her stuffed animals are all alone. And indeed, her stuffed animals were already very sad. The little brown teddy, her doll, the white rabbit Mr. Schlappohr and her little pink unicorn were all alone. Of course, that had to be changed immediately.

As Mama was packing laundry in the bedroom, Lydia scurried past her. The stuffed animals in her arms. Lydia placed the cuddly toys on Mom's and Dad's bed and said, "Problem solved." Then she rubbed her hands like daddy when he finished something.

Mama did not have that in mind when she told Lydia about the sad stuffed animals. She knelt down in front of Lydia and said, "My angel. Thats not OK. So we do not have enough space in the bed. We can hardly sleep that way."

Lydia thought for a moment. That's right, there was another problem. Mom and Dad were always too tired. Should she try to sleep in her own bed? Discouraged, she breathed out, "Phew. You and Dad are so far away. "She said. Mom looked at Lydia, "You mean when you sleep in your bed?" "Yes!" Lydia answered.

Now Mom thought, "Hm." Then she said, "What do you think if we leave your door a bit open. And we also leave ours a bit open. Then we'll hear you immediately, if anything should be. "

Lydia looked incredulous. But mom had an idea. "We'll try that out right away. That will be fun. What do you say? "Lydia nodded and ran to her room," Hello Mom! "She exclaimed. And mom answered, "Hello Lydia, my angel!" It actually worked. Lydia could hear Mama without Mom having to scream. So the two spent a while and made all sorts of funny sounds that the other had to guess.

When Dad came home, he went with him immediately. Now Mama called from the bedroom, Lydia from the nursery and dad from the room. That was funny. But dad had also brought two surprises.

Once a totally cuddly blanket and a great nightlight. The blanket was pink. Because Lydia loves pink. There were also little flowers on it, which almost looked like starlets. Asterisks would have preferred Lydia, but the flowers glowed in the dark and that was great.

The nightlight actually made little stars. If you turned it on, there were little glowing stars all over the nursery. When Dad said that the night light is extra for the night and allowed to stay all night, Mama immediately said, "Well, you see. Not only can you hear us, you can see everything in your room at night."

Now Lydia liked her room a lot better. And mom also had some news. Because if Lydia slept in her own bed now, then she was already big and brave. That's why Lydia was allowed to stay awake 15 minutes longer every evening. Lydia was happy and she felt really grown up.

After supper Lydia got ready for bed. From the bathroom she marched straight into Mom's and Dad's bedroom. What was going on now? Lydia wanted to sleep in her own bed today. Oh well, the stuffed animals were still there. Well, they had to be fetched, of course.

Then Lydia cuddled up with the new blanket in her cot. Teddy, Mr. Schlappohr, her doll and her unicorn around. The great nightlight sparkled and Mama read her another story. This Lydia could fall asleep really nice. She was sound asleep. And she even dreamed something nice.

CHAPTER 4

The Blue Kingfisher

Eight-year-old Jessica lived with her parents near a footpath. This snaked along a branch of the river. On Sundays people drove on it with the rowboat for a walk. They enjoyed the weeping willows and giant trees that dipped low over the river.

It was shady on the riverbank, quiet and mysterious. Jessica was not allowed to go near the shore alone - but sometimes she did. There was a blue bench standing on a small peninsula on the riverbank. She sometimes went there on Sunday mornings to watch Canada geese. The girl just sat there, watching those wonderful birds gather in droves and hear their loud chatter. Jessica thought this was a place full of magic. She was all alone with the geese. Jessica imagined that piece of forest by the river was hers alone. But of course we humans are only guests in nature. It belongs to itself. And it is full of miracles.

One morning, while the parents were still asleep, Jessica was sitting on her bench by the river again, waiting for the geese. But they did not come that morning. Instead, a small blue kingfisher came. He sat down on one of the branches on the edge of the water. Jessica hardly dared to breathe, so pretty was the little bird with its orange-yellow tummy and the bright blue plumage. She had never seen such a beautiful bird before. Suddenly the little kingfisher shot into the water. He soon reappeared with a small fish in his beak. Jessica behaved as quiet as a mouse. The bright blue bird flew back to the branch he had been sitting on and ate his fish. After that, he sat quietly on his branch for a while. He seemed to sleep. Suddenly a branch cracked somewhere and the shy bird flew away.

Jessica quickly walked home to tell her parents about this wonderful experience. Of course, the two scolded, because they were already worried. Little girls are not allowed to go to a river alone. But that Jessica loved nature so much, the parents could understand well.

Sleep-travel 33: The ticklish canoe

Far away in America, there lives the little Indian Pintu with his parents in a colorful Indian tent.

Today is Pintu's birthday. "You are already a big boy. That's why you get your own canoe, "says Pintu's father.

Pintu is very happy. He was allowed to ride with the adults, and even row. But the adults' canoes were far too big for him and hard to steer.

His own canoe is just right. It is smaller than an adult canoe and much more colorful and fun painted.

Pintu grabs his new canoe and runs down to the river. Pintu's mother is worried. "What if the river's current is too strong and the waves are too high?" "Do not worry, it's a very special canoe, nothing can happen to it!" Laughs Pintu's father.

Down the river, Pintu wants to let the canoe into the water. The river is very restless and wild at this point, but Pintu feels brave.

As he lets the canoe into the water, it suddenly starts to jump and giggle, so Pintu can not get in. "What's going on?" Asks Pintu. "I'm so ticklish, I can not be in the water with strong currents and high waves. Get me out! "Says the canoe. Pintu wonders. A canoe that can speak and is ticklish? What should he do with a ticklish canoe? "Let me into the water in a quiet place." Suggest the canoe. "The currents and waves do not tickle me and it's safer for you." Pintu likes the idea. He takes the canoe and leaves it in a quiet place in the water. Here the canoe does not jump and chuckle. Pintu can get in and both paddle happily on the river. If the water wilder, the small canoe does not continue, because it is far too ticklish.

Pintu's parents do not have to worry about Pintu being in danger.

CHAPTER 5

The Magic Book

Outside, a terrible storm was raging. Sonja lay bored on the bed. She leafed through a storybook. It was a birthday present from her aunt. After a while she fell asleep slowly. When she woke up, Sonja found herself on a lush green field. Confused, she stood up. How had she come here? Feverishly she thought about what to do now. Since she was a stranger to the area, she just ran in one direction. At first, Sonja saw nothing except many tall trees and shrubs.

The girl did not want to be beaten. She was a brave child after all. She would simply seek help. Somebody had to be here somewhere.

She continued for a while and finally came to a small house. White steam rose from the chimney. The enticing scent of cinnamon buns spilled out of the cracks in the window.

Tentatively, Sonja knocked on the door. Almost immediately, this was opened. An old woman with snow-white hair and very red cheeks behind. "Hello," Sonja said uncertainly. I was probably lost. Can you tell me how to find my way back to my room? - "Come in first," the woman replied cheerfully. "Have no fear. Here, try my fresh cinnamon rolls. It's just finished. "

Sonja sat down nicely at the table and bit into the pastry. It tasted heavenly. The dough was silky soft. The vanilla sugar melted on the tongue and the raisins made it very juicy. She was served warm cocoa. She ate until she was full. Then her eyes closed again.

The next time she woke up, she was surprisingly on bed again. Sonja realized that she had probably dreamed. She was about to slam the book when the old woman from the dream winked at her from one side.

CHAPTER 6

Mrs. Hexhex

Every day on the way to school and back again Olivia runs past a beautiful house where an old lady lives. Sometimes she sees her in the front yard, but she never says anything to her. The other children say that the old woman is a bad witch. One day, Olivia forgets her schoolbag in the school bus. But she not realizes it until she is almost in front of the old woman's house. "Oh no, shit!" Says Olivia when she realizes it. As always, the old lady is standing in her front yard. "What is it, my child?" She asks softly. Olivia answers politely what happened. "Maybe your dad can pick up the satchel at the nearest bus stop?"

But Olivia does not dare to tell her parents that she was so fussy and forgot her bag. "Hm," says the old woman. "Maybe I can help". "She? But you're a wicked witch ... "Olivia quickly puts her hand over her mouth. "I'm sorry, the other kids say that". The old woman just smiles. "I am the woman Hexhex. And you, what is your name? "" I am Olivia. You are not angry? "The old lady now giggles" No. Come in the front yard ". Olivia goes to her.

Mrs. Hexhex mumbles something and suddenly a broom comes flying. "Come on, get up," she says, helping Olivia climb the broom. The broom rises in the air and both fly high up. Olivia is excited "Mrs. Hexhex, where are we flying?". "Let yourself be surprised," she says and pushes the tube. Hui, that was a wind! After a few minutes they arrive at the next bus stop and land next to the bus. Olivia can bring her schoolbag and is happy. "Ms. Hexhex, you are a good witch and have helped me so much," she calls, back up in the air and shining all over her face.

CHAPTER 7

The Little Match Girl

The evening was horribly cold with mild wind and quite dark as it gently snowed; the last night to be experience before the next year. In this horrible weather, a poor girl walked along with no hoods on and on bare feet. It was obvious she had some shoes on before she left home, but how could she retain a large pair of shoes that was five times are shoe size; she had lost a leg of shoe in a mounted ridge of snow just across their rickety old house, as some horses hurried across with their carriages in very dreadfully fast.

Little Mary had lost a leg buried under the snow and the other pilled off her leg as she ran across. So the little poor girl scrabble her tiny bare feet on the freezing cold snow. Knowing she might not eat tomorrow without selling her box of matches, she struggled through as she hawked her matches; a couple of boxes in her torn, old apron and a few other in hand, this little industrious maiden walked door to door and not a soul gave her a dime for her matches.

Her concern wasn't really not making sales; but her freezing body and feeble fingers, as the snowflakes cover her soft blonde hair. As she walked pass the glowing windows of well-to-do families, she could perceive the delicious cakes and sweet savoury chickens as the candles and light stands spread its lights unto the streets of Compton. "It was New Year's Eve," she thought, and it was obvious she was going home to nothing but oddly prepared porridge.

At the end of the street, she found a small ledge to seat and huddled herself together; her tiny feet drawn very close to her face to help her keep warm before setting out to continue hawking. She knew there just was no need to go home without making any sales; it was not an option. She was almost accustomed to the cold as her corner was always very cold as well; she had a small blanket laid on the bare floor to rest on at night. He going home meant being spiked so had by her Dad, who is a Die-hard drunkard.

Freezing cold, her small arm was almost white with cold. She so wished she could light a match to herself to keep warm; it surely would do her a world of good at this point. She struck, as it kindled a small fire; it meant the world to her at this point. Tender and naïve as was, she stood it on the cold ice to keep warm and aimed to stretch her arms over the small fire; and obviously the tiny flame went out.

Earlier that week, Mr. Croak an old blacksmith had fallen off the horseback on his travel from the next town and Mary saved him. On this faithful day, Mary was dry cold near death. Unknowing to her she was leaning on the mayor's wall; she lighted another match stick to keep warm. Just then the mayor's wife saw a sparkle of light through the damp snowy window glass and reached out to open it. There she was little adorable Mary, cowed up to just sustain her warmth.

She beaconed on her to step into the house and draw warmness from the fireplace. Mary was served a warm bath and was given a sweet delicious goose prepared with the most amazing spices. It was then the Mayor's wife asked her why she was out with no guidance or nothing to keep her warm.

In tears, she narrated her ordeal on how she was passed to a careless and abusive drunkard step-dad and the fact the she had lost her both parents. The Mayor's wife was so embittered and invited the man the next day.

Finally, Mary was adopted by the mayor and she was given the finest things money can buy. However, she never missed to help her new mother keep to every normal chore that needed done before she takes off to school early in the morning.

Moral lesson

Do well to people, because it might not really be repaid by the same persons; but one way or another we all need help at some point in our lives.

The Kingdom Of Light

Long time ago, in a fine Glowing City live Lesley and Fabio who where brothers and lived together in a small house in their parents farm, it was a nicely crafted house they built together alittle far from the lively town of Kadibo. As fun and peaceful as they were trained, they did almost everything together; sleeping, eating, playing and even farming as well.

Their play time was the most amazing time for them as they played at any given time they wanted to; Moon light or sun.

They will bask in the sands as the sun rayed down on them, sight the stars as they shine their lights together and swirl around as the moon glommed. The brothers were everywhere around the farm together, chasing beams of light as the days broke and went down. It was obvious they never loved themselves any less and was always ready to do things together to achieve one single goal.

It was not enough to just love themselves. They wanted to love themselves for eternity as they continued their chase on light beams. So they decided to visit the Glowing King to help them seal their wish of being together forever.

It was a far journey into town to see the King as they sojourned along the lonely path into the king's palace. As they entered the city hall; on a magnificent throne sat a Glowing figure, sparkling like a thousand stars and having the brightness of the sun. They could barely see him lights from him damped their sight; with his feet soaked in beams of light.

Unguided they matched to the foot of the high throne and knelt down. "Why have you come?" The King asked. In fear and trembling they answered unanimously, "We have come to ask for your favour O King!" "We would love to request that you help use stay together and live happily."

The king was amazed at their zeal, even as peasants and granted their request. "Two shall do more wonders than one the zealous shall ripe their labour," he conjured. "For your determination and devotion, you will walk in a new light and join in the glow of a new done."

And he blessed them and the brothers set back to their lonely but happy peasant life in their small farm.

Days past with their regular life of farming and enjoying the chase of light beams at their leisure and nothing much happened.

One morning, as Fabio left early in the morning to pick woods in the forest, he saw a fine fig fruit and loved it; up he went to pluck it and hence from the top of the tree he saw a sparkling light from a spot just across the lake beside the farm. He was certain it was a gem and out of joy made his way home to break the news to his brother.

On getting to their apartment, he saw the house wide open. As he approached, he pondered, "Why would the door be open?" Still skeptical, he entered the house with no trace of Lesley anywhere in the house.

He was worried as he searched for Lesley with no trace. He called out his name severally, but no response as he wondered path into the apartment from the woods. "Maybe he went shopping for comic books," he thought, looking back at intervals.

Then he thought of walking back into the forest, after a tedious and confusing walk back into the forest, he saw a bright light far into the woods and decided to follow.

As he drew closer, he saw Lesley jumping around in excitement; with a mixed feeling of joy and weariness, as they celebrated their new found home a cave filled with precious stones and all manner of amazing gems. They will always be happy together and wealthy as they keep loving themselves.

They called for a banquet and invited the king as well as the townsmen, wherein they advised them on the importance of focusing their goals and loving one another.

Moral lesson

Never give on what you seek, you will definitely find it one day. Also, love is the best way to stay happy and live longer; it takes nothing to care about others.

CHAPTER 8

The Naughty Boy

Once upon a time, there lived a simple and just old poet. He loved to seat in front of his house and guise at the sky as the sun goes down. One beautiful evening as he sat outside rumbling from a distance was a great storm and accompanied by lightening and then rain. He hurried in and sat by his fireplace as he made fire and gazed at it as the flame burnt up.

Deep in thought he puzzled, "O the homeless would be soaking wet by now!" "I wish I had a lot I could do with my feeble hands to help."

Clak!! Clak!! Clak!! He had a gentle and mild knock on his door; it sounded so soft that he could identify it was a kid from the distance he sat. "Please let me in, I'm very cold." The child said, in a very faint voice.

As the old poet opened the door, he saw the little boy standing so cold and wet; and stared so seriously at him. "O Poor boy!" he exclaimed. "He really would be freezing cold in this rumbling tempest.

"Come in my boy," he said, as the old boy took the little fellow by hand into his apartment. He offered him a hot tea and some slices of bread to keep him warm as they sat together beside the fireplace. From all indication the little boy had gone deer hunting by himself before the storm met him in the jungle. He had a small bow with some arrows arranged in fine style to give him a fine hunter outlook even in his damp state.

The both sat in front of the fireplace as the flame died down the little boy got warm by time. He helped him dry quickly by giving him a heavy blanket to clean up as he drank his hot tea. With time he recovered and bounced back on his feet.

"What is your name young man," the old poet asked "and what took you out into this frightening storm.

“I’m Java he said and it is not nice to ask a stranger his name.” The little boy say so bold and firm on his feet. “I would love to take my leave sir.”

“O boy!” said the old poet, “you are not fully dry and bow is still wet.”

“That is a pity” the boy said, picking up his bow and an arrow. At this stance, he took a clear aim at the old poet and shot him on his shoulder. “O you can see old man, my bow is quite dry!” he said.

The old poet yelled and called on neighbours as the boy made his way out through the door. At this point he could count on all the good deeds he meted on little Java. He was taken in for medical care, but vowed to be careful when dealing with strangers in the future.

Moral lesson

Sometimes the people we want to save don’t deserve to be saved.

CHAPTER 9

The Green Orc

Once upon the time, there lived a King, who once had a lot of children and she lost them all to death but just one, a daughter. And she loved her so much, not just that she was so beautiful and fun to be with; she was the fairest of all in the city. Years passed and the King was growing old and need to carry her grand children, but she never wanted to get married. Advises fell on deaf ears as the King engaged her to please get married every day.

One day she decided to consult the a great wizard over the seven seas and seven mountains; she travelled with the finest men she could sort in her army. But all of them were mysteriously killed. Weary and feeble the old King huddled through the last test to the home of the wizard far inside the forbidden forest.

As he approached he was stopped by two scary pythons, raging with fury and ready to swallow him. Filled with fear and weak to his bones he managed to draw his sword but could barely do anything. In his weakness he saw a little green Orc.

"O King!," the Green Orc exclaimed. "Promise to hand your fair daughter, the princess to me if I save thy."

The king in fear hastened to accept his proposal and the Orc forced the pythons off as he fiercely fought them off. The path was cleared and the king went in to consult with the wizard on the fate of her beautiful daughter.

"She will marry her best fit." said the Wizard. "Go and worry not!"

And the King left and in joy. Days turned to weeks and weeks to months and no suitor had visited the palace to ask after the beautiful princess.

Then finally on a faithful day as the king won a great battle, and called a banquet of all the provinces under his rule; then the princess met a charming prince of the warrior clam of the city.

They fell in love and as time passed proposed marriage to the king. Filled with joy the king approved and fixed a date for the great feast. In few weeks, everything was set to take place as the princess was the ready to marry the prince.

On the wedding day, as the prince was get to receive her bride and all noble guest and kings for kingdoms far and near sat diligently to witness the wedding of the fairest lady in the kingdom. Just before the princess stepped unto the stump; the Green Orc in the totality of his ugliness.

“O king!” he exclaimed, “you had promised me your daughter in marriage, here I am to receive her as my wife.” Filled will fury and anger the king stood, eyes glaring red and burning to his bones. He ordered the arrest of the green Orc. Just before his soldiers could lay hold on the Orc, the princess fell, lifeless and cold as death.

The whole congregation thrown into panic and chaos, the king called for all the prominent physicians of the land, but known could heal her. Then the great wizard of the seven seas and seven mountains was summoned.

“You made a great promise my king.” he said “and it is time to fulfill your promise to my good friend the orc.” In tears and regretting why he could make such a hasty choice for her only daughter, he accepted all over again to give out her daughter to the Green orc as wife. Immediately, the princess came back to life. Finally the princess was married to the Green orc and taken to a kingdom far away from the city.

Moral lesson

Don’t make hasty choices, think about your decisions before concluding on anything

CHAPTER 10

The fearless Willbi

There used to be a little mouse in Africa. She lived in a small village on the edge of the jungle. In Africa it was very hot and in the village where the mouse lived there was no waterhole, no lake or even a small pond nearby. "Phew," the mouse snorted. "I have to get out of here." Said, done and so the mouse decided to visit her brother in the jungle.

There were many waterholes in the jungle. In her mind, the mouse was already swimming in the cool water and a smile crossed her face. "Brrrrr, the water is pretty cool." She thought. Quickly the bathing trunks packed into a small suitcase and off we went.

When she arrived in the jungle with her brother, the little mouse wondered about the house. All windows were tight and light was burning inside. The mouse knocked. Inside it rumbled and then it was quiet. The mouse knocked again: "Hey!" She called. "I heard you. Now get on Jonas! "The door opened a little gap. First there was a sniffing nose, then the blinking of small eyes.

Jonas threw open the door and jumped into his brother's arms, "Oh, Willbi. You are s. That's nice to see you. "Then Jonas looked around left and right. "Okay, come in quickly," he said and closed the door. Willbi looked around. Everything was pretty dark. "Why do you have the windows ... oh no," said Willbi. "I am here for a beach holiday! Nobody can handle the heat! So, grab your swimsuit and off you go! "

Jonas looked at Willbi anxiously, "You want to go swimming? To the water hole? But Willbi, that's where all the animals go. It's dangerous in the jungle! "" Excuse me? Pappalapapp, come on! "Jonas tugged on Willbi's arm:" No Willbi - really - it's too dangerous. So many animals are stronger than us and want to eat us. "But Willbi was not deterred. "If you do not pack your swimsuit, I'll do it!" He said, pulling Jonas after him.

The first thing they encountered was a lion. "Ahhh!" Yelled Jonas and scurried behind Willbi. Willbi looked at the lion. "What? Are you afraid of that? "Then he pulled his ears apart, stuck out his tongue, and made:" Bölölölölölöl. "But the lion just looked at him bored. "What?" Said Willbi. "You are not afraid of me?" The lion smiled tiredly: "I am the king of the jungle; why should I be afraid of a little mouse like you? "

"What, little mouse?" Said Willbi, pulling up his sleeves. "You're pretty naughty for such a hairy litter cat." Jonas tugged on Willbis shirt: "Listen to Willbi. He's much taller than us. "But Willbi waved his hand." Oh, pappalapap. People run away when I do that. Who really believes who he is? "

The lion looked at Willbi in amazement: "The people are afraid of you?" Willbi plumped proudly: "And whether! They jump on chairs and tables - if they see me! "The lion laughed loudly. Then he took a deep breath and yelled in the direction of the mice. Willbis ears fluttered in the wind of roar. It was so loud that all the birds nearby were startled and flying away.

But Willbi was unimpressed: "Pah, was that all? You should brush your teeth again! "Now the lion was startled. With a thoughtful look, he studied Willbi again. "You are not afraid of me? he asked. "Nope!" Willbi said firmly. "Why should I? You should be afraid of me! "

The lion did not really know what was happening. There was a small mouse with rolled-up sleeves in front of him, looking at him angrily. "You say: people are afraid of you? Prove it! "The lion finally said. "Pah." Willbi said. "No problem!"

They sneaked into the nearby village. The lion was afraid of humans and stopped more often the closer they came to the village. "What's wrong? Did the courage leave you? "Willbi called cheekily." "The little mouse really does not seem to be afraid," thought the lion.

When he arrived in the village, Willbi said: "Okay, Pussycat. You look through the window. I go in and show you how to deal with people. Jonas, you stay with the rental cat. "" What? "Jonas asked. "But he's eating me." "Oh, my," said Willbi. "The Mietze is not afraid of hunger." And went into the house.

The lion did not believe his eyes when he saw people jumping over tables and benches when they saw the little mouse. Willbi ran back and forth and made his face: "Bölölölölö". Then he came out again: "Na Mietzi? Now you, "he said. But the lion was too scared. And so they sneaked back into the jungle.

At the waterhole, Willbi jumped directly into the cool water: "Juhuuu!" - Splash - Other animals gathered around the waterhole when they saw the mice, but they did not dare, because the big lion stood there. Hyenas, Jackals, Wildcats ... everyone was waiting for their chance.

When the lion saw that, he just said, "Keep calm. Attack the mice - I will not stop you. "The hyenas were looking forward to a delicious snack. "But be warned," said the lion further. "I would not do it. These are the strongest mice I have ever seen. All humans have fled from them. I've watched it with my own eyes! "

The other animals were confused and looked questioningly at. A hyena lisped, "Alas, if the lion does not even eat it, I'll leave it." Another hyena stuttered back, "Well, there you are. If the lion d does not do that mmm ma, I will not do it either.

Willbi swam on his back through the waterhole and trumpeted: "What's going on? Just dare. You will experience your blue miracle! "But the animals slowly crept away. They were too scared of the mice - even people were afraid of them.

And even after Willbi had driven back to the village on the edge of the jungle, no one dared approach Jonas. He no longer hid himself, let in the bright sunlight through all the windows, and lived happily ever after.

Sleep journey 15: The strange girl

One day a new girl came to kindergarten. Everybody thought her strange because she spoke only in rhymes. "Why are you talking so weird?" Little Marla asked the girl. The girl replied, "I'm not talking funny, that would be awesome. Almost astronomical and somehow stupid. "Then she went on. Marla stood with her mouth open: "Astro ... what?" She asked - but the girl was already out of earshot.

The more the girl spoke, the more children began to speak in rhymes. "Hello, kindergarten teacher, I have something in mind. I would like to have another tea. Would that be okay?"

The kindergarten teachers wondered about the children, who now only spoke in rhymes, but they also found it funny. And so they made themselves: "Hello dear children, we play a game now. The things of the inventor. Winning is the goal. "

It was not long before everyone in kindergarten spoke only in rhymes. When the parents picked up their children, they were very surprised that everything rhymed with what their children said: "We were almost only outside, I could barely catch my breath. It was so much fun. I did not think about the time. Now you are here and pick me up, can I still play short and sweet? "

The parents thought that was weird. Marla's mom asked Marla why she was talking so funny. Marla replied, "I'm not talking funny, that would be awesome. Almost astronomical and somehow stupid. "Marla's mom stood with her mouth open:" Astro ... what? "She asked - but Marla was already out of earshot.

The parents looked at each other in bewilderment. But then they began to rhyme themselves without realizing: "I see my child playing there. One among many. But it talks in rhymes. Will that stay that way? "Another mother turned around:" I can not say that, at least I do not believe it. But you too were talking in rhymes right now - almost like a poem. "Then everybody laughed.

Now a father intervened: "What should I tell my wife when she hears the child talking? I do not want to complain, but I'm a bit confused. "" You say that's normal - it's all rhyming now. If it were not so, then it would be fatal, because then it would be strange child. "

And so the parents began to rhyme. Then the parents' friends and it was not long before the whole country rhymed and those who did not rhyme were strange.

One day a strange girl came to kindergarten. It spoke without rhyming. Marla came and said: "You talk so funny. That's tremendous. Almost astronomical and somehow stupid. "

The strange girl asked in astonishment: "Astro ... what?" Marla looked at her: "I do not know what that means, but it sounds great," Marla said and shrugged her shoulders. Then the strange girl smiled and said, "I'm Luisa. Do you want to be my girlfriend, even if not everything rhymes what I say? "Marla thought for a moment. Then she took Luisa by the hand and said, "Sure! Let's play. I'll show you our great play area. "

And so the children gradually stopped rhyming. Then the kindergarten teachers stopped rhyming. Then the parents, the friends of the parents and soon the whole country.

And what do we learn from history? So it becomes strangely normal and normal becomes strange. But no matter how you are, it's as good as it is.

CHAPTER 11

The Bonded Donkey

This Short Story The Bonded Donkey is very intriguing to every one of the individuals. Appreciate perusing this story.

In a little town, there carried on a potter. He had a jackass. Regular his jackass would convey soil from the field to his home. Since the field was very distant, the potter would rest under a tree halfway, tying his jackass close by.

At some point, the potter neglected to take the rope with which he tied the jackass regular. When he arrived at the tree, he figured, "How would I tie this jackass today? He may flee on the off chance that I rest. "The potter chose to secure holding the jackass' ears with the goal that the jackass would not flee.

Be that as it may, thusly neither the jackass was agreeable nor the potter had the option to take rest. A holy person, who happened to be cruising by, saw the potter clutching the jackass' ears. At that point the holy person needed to recognize what the issue of the potter was. At the point when the potter told the holy person what the issue was, the savvy holy person stated, "Take thc jackass to where you tie him ordinary. Claim to tie him utilizing a fanciful rope. I guarantee you he won't flee." The potter did what the holy person had said.

He left the jackass and went to sleep. At the point when he woke up, incredibly and help, he found the jackass remaining in a similar spot.

Before long the potter arranged to leave for home. Be that as it may, the jackass didn't move. "What's going on with this jackass!" shouted the potter in dissatisfaction.

Fortunately, the potter saw the astute holy person once more. He approached the holy person and enlightened him concerning the jackass' peculiar conduct. The holy person stated, "You tied up the jackass, however did you unfasten him?" Go and claim to loosen the rope with which you had tied the jackass." The potter pursued the holy person's recommendation.

Presently the jackass was prepared to leave for home. The potter comprehended that jackass was the reinforced jackass. The potter expressed gratitude toward the shrewd holy person and returned home joyfully with his jackass.

Best Bedtime Stories for Children

Kids are constantly dynamic, and it tends to be difficult to put them to rest on occasion. This is the point at which a decent story can go to your guide. It causes you set up your children for sleep time, and they'll even anticipate it if there are great stories to hear. The following, are a portion of the accounts that you could peruse out to them.

1. The Ugly Duckling

Odd one out

This is one of the exemplary sleep time stories for kids. The story begins a ranch, where a duck sits on a grip of eggs to make them incubate. The eggs incubate individually, and soon, there are six yellow-feathered ducklings, twittering enthusiastically. The last egg takes more time to bring forth, and from it develops a weird looking duckling with dark quills. Everyone finds the dark duckling monstrous, including its very own mom. The down and out duckling flees and lives alone in a bog until winter comes. Seeing the duckling starving in winter, a rancher has compassion for the odd one out and gives it nourishment and safe house at home. Be that as it may, the duckling fears the rancher's boisterous kids and escapes to a cavern by a solidified lake. When spring comes, a group of wonderful swans dive on the lake, and the duckling, which is presently completely developed, however forlorn, approaches the swans, completely hoping to be dismissed. Shockingly, the swans invite him. He takes a gander at his appearance in the water and understands that he isn't an odd one out any longer, however a wonderful swan. The swan joins this run and takes off with his new family.

2. Midas and the Golden touch

Midas and the Golden touch

The account of Midas is another exemplary sleep time story for kids. This old story from Greece depicts King Midas as an eager and unhappy man, who adored gold more than all else. Once, he carried out something beneficial for somebody, and a Greek God showed up before him, saying that he will be allowed his deepest longing for carrying out the beneficial thing. Midas wanted that all that he contacted should transform into gold, immediately. The God conceded his desire. Midas was energized and approached contacting irregular articles, transforming all that he contacted into gold. Sooner or later, he got eager. In any case, when he contacted his nourishment, it went to gold, and he couldn't eat it. He was starving and unnerved that he couldn't eat. Seeing him agitated, his caring little girl tossed her arms around him to comfort him, and she, as well, went to gold. Midas was sickened that his girl had become a statue of gold. He lamented requesting the Golden Touch and understood that he had been insatiable and that gold was not the most valuable thing on the planet. He cried and asked the God to reclaim his desire. The God had compassion for him and requested that he take a plunge in the waterway by his royal residence, and afterward fill a pitcher of water from the stream and sprinkle it on every one of the things he needed to change back. He adhered to the directions and changed his little girl back to ordinary. He was exceptionally glad to recover his adored little girl and quit being covetous from that minute.

3. The Boy Who Cried Wolf

The Boy Who Cried Wolf

This story is from Aesop's Fables and intrigues the significance of being honest. It is the tale of a shepherd kid who watched a herd of sheep close to his town. The region was known to have a wolf that was scandalous for attacking the sheep run and carrying off several sheep. Each resident knew about the hazard and was constantly prepared to go to the guide of any individual who had an issue with the wolf. Be that as it may, the kid neglected this supportive nature of the locals, and truth be told, disparaged it. For his entertainment, he drew out the locals, multiple times, by shouting out for help, saying "Wolf! Wolf!". The ever-cautious townspeople promptly came to support him, just to discover the shepherd kid having a healthy giggle. They were normally disturbed when he snickered at them for getting tricked. At some point, in any case, a wolf really came and began executing and eating his sheep. This time, when he weeped for help, none of the residents went to his guide, as they thought he was pulling a trick on them once more. Subsequently, the wolf annihilated the shepherd's rush. The lesson of the story is that nobody accepts a liar, in any event, when he comes clean.

4. The Ant and the Grasshopper

Subterranean insect and the Grasshopper

This is another story from Aesop's Fables, and discusses the significance of difficult work and getting ready for what's to come. The story recounts a grasshopper that spends the mid year singing and sitting ceaselessly his time. In the interim, his neighbors, a settlement of ants, buckle down all through the late spring to store nourishment for the winter. The grasshopper giggles at the ants and discloses to them that they ought to appreciate the mid year. The ants tell the grasshopper that he should store nourishment for the winter or he will starve when everything is solidified. At the point when winter comes, the ants are in their home, laying and making due on the nourishment that they put away. The grasshopper goes to their entryway, ravenous and cold. He asks the ants for nourishment and says he understood the mistake of his ways. The ants share their nourishment with him and make him guarantee to buckle down, the following summer, to assemble and store nourishment.

5. Magnificence and the Beast

Magnificence and the Beast

This is a celebrated fantasy that discloses to us that we should look past outward appearances and give more significance to an individual's benevolence. There used to be a dealer who lost all sense of direction in a tempest and took cover in a palace that he found. While leaving, he culled a rose from the nursery to blessing to his little girl Belle. The stronghold had a place with a repulsive monster, who detained the shipper for attempting to take the rose. The dealer asked to be liberated and told the brute he just needed the rose for his little girl Belle. The Beast let him go, relying on the prerequisite that his little girl will have his spot and live in the stronghold. The dealer came all the way back and told Belle everything. Beauty went to live in the manor with the Beast, instead of her dad. The Beast experienced passionate feelings for the delightful Belle, who understood that the Beast was generally excellent natured and not horrendous. At some point, Belle requested that authorization go see her dad. At the point when she left, the Beast felt grief stricken. Beauty came back to the château, to see that the Beast was biting the dust. She held the Beast and cried, conceding that she adores him. Out of the blue, the Beast transformed into an attractive ruler. He was reviled by a witch that he would stay a Beast, until a lady genuinely cherished him, notwithstanding his ghastly looks. At the point when Belle said she adored the mammoth, the witch's revile was broken. The ruler and Belle got hitched and lived cheerfully ever after.

6. Cinderella

Cinderella

Cinderella is another fantasy brimming with enchantment and experience. Once, an excellent young lady named Cinderella lived with her insidious stepmother and two stepsisters. The stepmother caused her to do all the housework and was extremely merciless to her. At some point, the stepmother and stepsisters went to a ball in the King's castle, abandoning Cinderella. Cinderella truly needed to go to the ball and felt tragic that she had been deserted. All of a sudden, a pixie adoptive parent showed up in an explosion of light, and she utilized her enchantment to change Cinderella into a princess, wearing a flawless dress and glass shoes. She likewise transformed a pumpkin and a few mice into a carriage and steeds, separately. Cinderella could now go to the ball. The pixie adoptive parent cautioned her that the enchantment will wear off at 12 PM and that Cinderella should come all the way back before that. At the point when Cinderella landed at the ball, the sovereign saw her, and they experienced passionate feelings for. They moved together until late. At the point when the clock struck twelve, Cinderella raced to her carriage, departing one of her glass shoes behind. The sovereign scanned each house around the local area for the strange young lady whose foot fit into the glass shoe. He arrived at the underhanded stepmother's home and found that the shoe had a place with Cinderella. Subsequently, the sovereign and Cinderella got hitched and lived joyfully ever after.

7. The Hungry Mouse

The Hungry Mouse

This is among the short sleep time stories for kids. It discusses how insatiability can get individuals into terrible circumstances. There used to be a mouse that was starving and had not eaten in days. He had become truly slight. After a ton of looking, the mouse found a bushel loaded with corn. There was a small opening in the container, through which he could simply fit in. In this way, he crawled into the container and ate his fill of corn. Be that as it may, he didn't quit eating, when he was full. The mouse ate to an ever increasing extent, despite the fact that he was feeling full. Presently, the mouse had become bigger from such nourishment and could never again fit through the gap to get out. He was stressed and thought about how to get away. A rodent that was passing by heard the mouse and revealed to him that he needed to hold up until he had become slim once more, so as to get out through that opening. The mouse lamented being voracious and gorging.

8. I'm Bored

I am Bored

This is another short sleep time story for kids. The story is about a young lady who cries about weariness until she meets a potato. The potato reveals to her that children are exhausting. The young lady is astounded and tells the potato that children are not exhausting, and are in reality a great deal of fun. The potato requests that the young lady demonstrate this. The young lady tells the potato every one of the things kids do to have a fabulous time. She tells the potato that children can mess around, do cartwheels, skip, stroll on their hands, have a race, and play on the swing. She likewise tells the potato that superior to everything else, children can envision. This story is an approach to help kids to remember all the fun things they can do when they are exhausted. This story can likewise be intelligent in the event that you request that your kid relate all the fun things that he/she gets a kick out of the chance to do.

9. The Emperor's New Clothes

Ruler's New Clothes

This is an interesting sleep time story for kids. A glad and pretentious ruler just thinks about showing himself in excellent garments and delicacy. He contracts two weavers and guarantees them a prize in the event that they make for him the best suit of garments at any point worn by anybody.

5 of the best sleep time stories for adults to get you to rest

Rest Stories could be the appropriate response – a component of reflection application, Calm.

"There's a Catch 22 to rest, in that it comes when no doubt about it", he says. "At the point when you attempt to rest, your mind screens your endeavors, which at that point keeps you conscious. Rather, have the expectation of unwinding and giving up.

"The initial phase in getting a decent night's rest is being in the correct mentality. In case you're drained, loose and prepared for rest you will consequently nod off following 10 to 20 minutes. This is the reason accomplishing something quieting before bed will help set you up for rest.

This can be contemplation, perusing (nothing excessively energizing) or now tuning in to a 'Rest Story', intended to assist you with giving up and slide into a quiet sleep."

Quiet fellow benefactor Alex Tew includes: "Recollect when you were youthful the amount you delighted in tuning in to a sleep time story? It was consoling, unwinding and mitigating.

"At the point when you're a youngster, you have considerably less at the forefront of your thoughts and rest comes effectively. Rest Stories are intended to return you to a less complex mental state and let your mind unwind and plan for a profound rest, similarly as it did when you were youthful. There's no explanation we can't all have a decent night's rest... without drug."

CHAPTER 12

Kyoto

Our visit to Japan includes a tour of the many temples, shrines, and palaces in Kyoto, the cultural center of Japan. Home to thousands of significant spiritual sites scattered across the valley formed by mountains on three sides of the region. With so many places to experience, it would be hard to see everything in a few days, so we start with one of the most loved sites in the area, the Fushimi Inari-Taisha shrine. A Shinto shrine that winds through a lush forest, up a mountain path while taking us through thousands of vermillion red Torii gates placed close together. In the Shinto religion, these gates signify the transition of the mundane to the sacred. Knowing this, it feels as though each step brings you closer to something magical, and with the walk being over 3 miles, we enjoyed this feeling of anticipation for hours.

We go early in the morning to avoid the crowds and began our walk through the first gate just as the sun was coming up. It's a brisk day in the small window between winter and spring when the trees start to come alive again. Across the region, budding blossoms of pink cherry trees are beginning to form. The path takes us up a small slope, and we are enveloped by Torii gates, creating a crimson tunnel up the mountain. After a short walk the tunnel lets us out into a clearing, there is a path that leads off the main trail to a small temple, and we take a short rest on the steps there. The forest and its temples are home to several stray cats, and we are greeted by curious felines. We watch them emerging from all directions to bask in the few sunbeams sneaking in through the treetops. We continue the walkthrough hundreds and hundreds of towering red gates in near silence. Feeling in awe of such a beautiful homage to the Shinto deities. From the top, we enjoy a view of the valley from the Inchinomin temple and begin the journey back down to the main gate.

Feeling tired from the morning hike, we decide to have an early lunch at one of the cafes and then enjoy a traditional tea ceremony to finish off the day. Fushimi Inari-Taisha shrine is dedicated to the gods of rice and sake, so it is fitting to enjoy a bit of both with our meal. The tea ceremony is a sacred tradition of Japan, and we are excited to participate fully in the experience. This particular location fully submerges us in the culture with our own Kimono and a full explanation of the tea ceremony. The friendly staff help us choose a Kimono for the occasion, mine is a bright blue with a pattern of vivid pink and green flowers. My hair is pulled up in a simple updo by the delicate hands of the workshop facilitators, and we are ready to enter the tearoom. We sit in the traditional style, on our knees facing our host, and we bow to each other as we settle in.

The tea ceremony begins with a tray placed in front of our host with the tools needed to serve us. Everything has a specific purpose, and the sequence of the ceremony honors all aspects as well as the esteemed guests. Our host takes us through the tea ceremony so we may have the experience, and then explains each step to us. Later we will try and make the tea ourselves. On the tray is a beautiful ceramic bowl, decorated on one side with vibrant red leaves, and the other is the unmistakable pattern of cherry blossoms on a branch. In the bowl is a bamboo whisk, a small white cloth, and a long silver spoon with the tiniest scoop delicately curved up from the end. The tray also contains a small black ceramic jar with a lid and another ceramic container painted in vibrant green. In front of the tray is a cast-iron kettle with a large arched handle placed on a square tile on the floor.

Our host begins her ceremony by bowing to us, and we bow in turn. She removes a folded square of red silk fabric from the belt in her Kimono. She folds it over itself several times with precision. Gracefully, with the folded silk cloth, she picks up the black jar with the painted lid and gently wipes one edge, then another. She places her hand on top of the jar and smoothly pulls her hand off and places the jar back on the tray. It is not spoken, but it is understood that she is purifying the contents, and we already feel incredibly honored.

Our host unfolds and refolds the red cloth and applies the same gentle precision to the long metal scoop, softly squeezing both the handle and the scoop. She places the scoop on the tray, removes the whisk and cloth from the decorated bowl, and reaches for the cast-iron kettle. She slowly pours steaming water into the bowl, using the cloth to protect her hands from the hot lid. With the whisk, she stirs the hot water around the edges of the bowl.

Inspecting the whisk as she works, she empties the water into the green bowl and uses the white cloth to wipe out the inside of the warmed bowl. We are entranced by the preciseness of her actions. When she bows to signify the completion of the purification, we almost miss our cue to bow back.

Our host removes the lid from the black jar to reveal a bright green powder. With her scoop, she adds two heaping piles of the powder to the bowl and gently places her tools back on the tray. She carefully adds hot water to the bowl. With the bamboo whisk, she quickly and skillfully whisks the tea into a creamy, frothy drink. Once the tea is prepared, she turns the bowl in her hands and places it in front of me so that the cherry blossom design faces me. I am the guest and receive instruction on how to accept this gift with the same grace it was made. I bow and say, "Thank you" in Japanese. I place the tea bowl in the palm of my left hand and cup it with the fingertips of my right hand, I raise the bowl up, in a symbol of gratitude. With my right hand, I turn the bowl twice. Now the cherry blossoms face our host. It is nearly spring, so we are honoring the coming season by placing significance on the blossoms. With both hands, I raise the bowl to my mouth and take in the fresh, earthy flavor of matcha tea. I consume the full serving in three sips, and when finished, wipe the edge of the bowl gently with two fingers. Using my special guest napkin provided with my Kimono. It was tucked in just the right spot for the occasion as I was helped into my Kimono. I turn the bowl again and pass the empty bowl back to my host.

To close the ceremony, our host rinses the bowl with more hot water, empties it in the larger green bowl, and we bow to each other. If I wished I could have another tea made for me, but it is everyone else's turn for the honor. Our host pours more water, rinses the whisk in the bowl, and empties it. She then assembles all of her tools back into the tea bowl. For each guest, the ceremony is repeated with care, and we sit in a respectful peace. We enjoy each moment for its simplicity, dedication, and pure mindfulness of the long-standing tradition of a cup of tea. As I watch my fellow guests enjoy the experience, I know I will be treating each cup of tea I make from now on with more reverence from now on.

CHAPTER 13

New Orleans

In some cities, the history of it is just something tourists come to see for a few days, but in New Orleans, history is part of everyday life, and the locals live in it full time. A still functioning piece of history is used every day to bring people about their lives and have done so for a hundred years. The one thing that lives up to this the most is the streetcars of New Orleans. In most cities, artifacts like streetcars are something the locals avoid. Stepping on a tram in New Orleans, you are as likely to sit beside a local musician as you would be to sit beside a tourist here to see some musicians play while in town.

For my trip through the many diverse neighborhoods of Nola, I start on the St. Charles line, the oldest running continuous streetcar in the world. For over 150 years, this olive-green streetcar has been rumbling through these streets. Taking people to and from work, play, and everything in between. The route forms a crescent through the Central Business District along Canal Street and into the prestigious Uptown neighborhood. I pay my fair of 1.25 in exact change as requested by the sign on the front of the car and take a window seat a few rows behind the operator. Inside, the seats are the original mahogany benches, and the brass fittings have stood the test of time. The operator uses a lever system to control the small wheels that the roomy streetcar is perched on. With the twist of their wrist, the car lurches into action. These were not built for aerodynamics or comfort. Still, the old-fashioned charm of the hundred-year-old public transportation quickly grows on me.

The car rocks side to side as it picks up speed toward the next station, and as it lumbers through the city, passengers hop on and off at the different stations. The track takes a sweeping turn at the curve of the crescent, and the driver effortlessly directs the large metal box on wheels around the bend and down the legendary St. Charles Avenue. Soon we're in the historic Uptown section of New Orleans. Here along the east bank of the mighty Mississippi river, we chug along the track through a long tunnel of oak tree branches. The trunks rooted in front yards of stately mansions that line parts of the street. The houses are from picture books and movies, emphasizing the charm and romance of Nola. Beautifully keep estates, with large front porches that sweep all the way around the side of the white or yellow home, with ornate columns that hold up the second-floor balcony.

The streetcar rocks its way through the old neighborhood picking up and dropping off locals and tourists alike. Near the end of the line, I jump off at a station across from a large white cathedral. It has arched doorways, spires on every peak, and a bell tower that reaches high above the leafy oak tree canopy. A few blocks down a few side streets, lined with more homes each with a unique charm but all within the same style of porches, columns, and balconies, there is a small cemetery with a large population, the Lafayette cemetery takes up only one city block but with its many family mausoleums is the final home of family members stretching back as far as the city's history does. The large stone structures, each with their own unique charm, remind me of the rows of stately homes I just passed on the streetcar and how we all want a little piece of beauty with us no matter where we are in life.

I wander the narrow paths noting how ferns grow from the cracks that have developed over time. Indicating that life will always find a way to spring forth from even the smallest of opportunities. The space has a somber effect, but the splashes of green reminds me that there is always hope and something to believe in. If these ferns can thrive here, in the forgotten cracks of history in New Orleans, then I imagine that any struggle I face is manageable if just persevere.

Leaving the cemetery, I hear a lively jazz band striking up, and I find my way to the bar they are playing in. The band is on a stage inside with a few people scattered about the room listening in, music is everywhere in this city, and I think it needs to be. Like the ferns in the cracks, New Orleans relies on the little glimmers of life. The streetcar still running after all these years. The old homes with porches that housed many families and played host to their triumphs and struggles. The jazz standards passed down from generation to generation. All of these have stood the test of time and wear layers of history like strands of beads around the necks of mardi gras participants, one-part beauty, one-part a weighty ache. I enter the bar and find a stool near the street to watch the band and the streetcar, both chugging forward with a rhythm that is uniquely New Orleans.

CHAPTER 14

LAKE OF INNER DISCOVERY

Steps for increasing effectiveness of the story:

1. What do you want to achieve from reading this?
2. Think about one thing you have achieved today.
3. Say to yourself "When I read this story then..."

Alternative introduction:

"As I read this and begin to drift comfortably asleep, I don't know whether I will find myself drifting asleep more to the sound of my voice or the words I read, or perhaps to the spaces between the words. And as I drift comfortably asleep I'll just read this story to myself."

As you listen to me you can begin to relax and you will relax as deeply and comfortably as you can right now. And as the experience goes on, so you will relax deeper and even more comfortably. To the point where, as you continue listening to this adult bedtime story, you will discover yourself falling asleep without even noticing. And you will continue the story perhaps in your dreams, or perhaps you will get through to near the end of the story and just drift off asleep, deeply and comfortably, getting the appropriate sleep through the night.

And so, as you continue listening to me I'm going to tell you a story where you are the main character and it can be a little bit like a lucid dream where you are aware of the story playing out around you, aware of what you can see, what you can hear, what you can feel.

And so you go on a journey one day and as you take this journey, you are walking out through the woods and while you walk through the woods, you are wondering about different things, you are wondering about what it is you have got to do later, you are wondering about a conversation you had earlier or the previous day, you are wondering about someone you are going to see later in the week and a part of you is also aware of, the sounds around you, is also aware of the feeling of each footstep you take as you walk through the woods, is also aware of the sounds of the rustling leaves and noticing the dancing light, as it shimmers through the trees.

And while you are out on this nice and relaxed walk, you are searching for a lake, you have never visited this lake before, you have been told that if you come out into this wood you can discover a lake, a lake that will help you find some inner discovery and you are curious what inner discovery you can get by finding this lake. So, as you are out walking around you notice rabbits hopping around, you notice birds flying, you notice butterflies and bees going about their daily business; popping in and out of different flowers.

And you don't know what kind of inner discovery you are going to gain at the lake and what it is about the lake that will help you find that inner discovery, you just know it is what you have been told. So, you walk along the path going deeper into the woods and as you go deeper and deeper into the woods, so you relax more with the experience, that kind of daydream relaxation that you have, as you are walking along, where your mind is wandering and feeling pleasant, where the day just feels so pleasant, that you just feel so relaxed. And while you wander along you hear someone down the path, so you keep walking, you are curious who that person is going to be and as you get closer you can hear their voice speaking louder.

And then as you approach you notice, a man dressed in nondescript clothing, a man who can just blend in anywhere, he even seemed to almost blend in here, if it wasn't for his talking. And because you are walking through the woods and there is only you and this man, it is only polite to say hello, as you walk past. And as you walk past and you say hello, so the man responds to you. "Do you know where you are going here in the middle of nowhere?" The man asks.

You think you understand what the man says as you experience a little confusion and you tell him yes you are trying to find the lake and he responds "Yes you are trying to find the lake and the lake is in the middle of nowhere and nowhere is where you are going and you will know where you are going when you discover that nowhere is here and here in the middle of nowhere is nowhere. And some people try to travel to somewhere and other people try to travel to anywhere, but you're not trying to go somewhere or anywhere, you are here nowhere and as you walk around here nowhere, you should be able to find the lake you are looking for. Because the lake you are looking for is nowhere, but in your mind." And with that the man began to walk away. And left you feeling a little confused.

And so, you continued to walk along the path looking for the lake and you didn't know where you were going exactly, but you knew that you would find the lake following this path. So you continued looking along the path, going deeper into the woods and as you relax deeper and deeper into the woods, so the, woods appear to, become thicker and denser and that made them become slightly darker, but that helped you to notice that as you turned a corner on the path, that there was a clearing off in the distance because it was much brighter over there and you didn't pick up the pace or speed up in anyway just because you noticed the clearing, but you now knew where you were going. You were confident that in that clearing, that you would find the lake that you were searching for. And as you are walking along towards that clearing, so you have the words of that man going around in your head. Nowhere, somewhere, anywhere. You thought to yourself quizzically. Nowhere, somewhere, anywhere.

You didn't know exactly what he was on about, but the same way when you meet someone and you can't remember their name but you know you know their name but the harder you try to remember their name, the harder it becomes to remember and then you just put it out of your mind and you carry on with other things and then their name springs up in your mind a little while later, you knew the same thing would probably happy here and if you just carry on with the journey and you put what that man said out of your mind and the answer will just spring up in mind when the time is right, there is no need to try and force it, the answers will come through when the unconscious has worked it out enough to let you know.

And as you approach the clearing you notice the most beautiful lake, such calm water and as you gaze across the lake the water is so calm that the reflection in the water is almost indistinguishable from what it is reflecting. And you are aware that if you took a photo and turned the photo upside-down people probably wouldn't be able to tell which one is the water and which one is the sky, which one is just the reflection.

And you had never seen a lake as still as this and you felt it was really odd that this lake should be so still given there was the most refreshing, beautiful breeze on your skin. Because you expect the breeze to move the water.

And as you approach the lake you can see a sign and so you walk over to the sign and on the sign, is some writing and the writing says 'pick up a stone and throw it in and watch how it sinks to the bottom and keep your eyes firmly fixed on the stone, don't be distracted by the ripples of the lake, don't be distracted by any other movement, don't be distracted by sounds, just keep your eyes focused on the stone as it hits the water and sinks to the bottom and keep your eyes focused on that stone and you will gain inner discovery.'

And then there was an arrow pointing down beneath the sign to some purple stones. And next to the purple stones was a small sign, saying 'pick the stone that feels right for you' and so you put your hand down and you feel the different stones and you can feel how some are rougher than others and you can see that some were matt and others are reflective and you can see how the stones are all different shapes and sizes. They all have different textures and so you feel the different stones in your fingertips, feeling the weight, the size, the shape, until you find one that feels right and comfortable for you.

And once you have found that comfortable stone you can throw it in the lake and you can let your eyes follow the stone through the air as it arches towards the lake. You let your eyes follow the stone to the surface, hearing that sound of the stone breaking the surface, seeing the splash of water, hearing the plop sound as the stone enters the lake and watching as the stone waves slightly left and right as it sinks to the bottom and as the sign said, you keep your eyes on the stone as it sinks to the bottom and while it is on the bottom you keep your eyes on the stone and you notice how the ripples begin to spread out from where the stone entered the water and as the ripples reach the shore, so the reeds by the bank begin to wave as they are knocked about by the water. And as the ripples travel across the lake so they spread out further and further. Spreading further apart as they travel across the lake and you followed the instructions, you have kept your eyes focused and fixed on that stone, out of your peripheral vision you can notice the movement and you don't let it bother you, you just keep your eyes fixed on the stone and after a few minutes the strangest thing can begin to happen. Your peripheral vision begins to go black and the stone begins to become even clearer and you begin to have a sense of clarity.

And then as the lake becomes still, you notice that between you and the stone is you and it is as if you are looking into your own eyes, looking into your own soul, looking into your heart. Seeing yourself for the first time. Not the self you normally see in a mirror, but your deeper self, your inner self. And so you can take some time of peace and silence, feeling a slight sense of excitement of your discovery, to begin to, gain that inner discovery, from the weird reflective nature of this lake and how that is somehow connected to a stone entering the lake, creating ripples yet everything becomes still like nothing has happened and yet you are aware something has happened, you are aware, something entered the lake and the lake is different to how it was before you arrived because of your actions and yet on the surface it looks no different, but deep down, something has changed and so you take some time to enjoy some silence to develop inner meaning and discovery.

And after a while, you feel you have been discovering something and learning something, deep inside your mind and so you begin to walk away from the lake. You now know where it is when you want to come back here again and so you walk away from the lake, back through the woods. And as you walk back through the woods so you walk deeper and deeper and drift deeper and deeper and fall asleep comfortably, easily and effortlessly. And you can take as long as you like to absorb yourself in the process of walking back through the woods and knowing unconsciously there is a lot that you have learned. And so, you can enjoy taking a nice leisurely stroll back through the woods, going deeper and more comfortably asleep.

CHAPTER 15

THE ASTRONAUT'S WONDER

Steps for increasing effectiveness of the story:

1. What do you want to achieve from reading this?
2. Think about one thing you have achieved today.
3. Say to yourself "When I read this story then..."

Alternative introduction:

"As I read this and begin to drift comfortably asleep, I don't know whether I will find myself drifting asleep more to the sound of my voice or the words I read, or perhaps to the spaces between the words. And as I drift comfortably asleep I'll just read this story to myself."

As you listen to this, so you will begin to fall asleep and you may fall asleep before the end of this or you may feel comfortably relaxed and drift off into a comfortable sleep at the end of this and as you listen to this, this also has useful therapeutic messages within this story and it's not a detailed story, it's purpose is to be a bit like drifting in a dream where you are playing the lead role, where it is something calming and comfortable, that helps you drift comfortably asleep.

So as you listen to me, you can begin to notice yourself as an astronaut. You are walking along towards a giant rocket and you have got some astronaut crew with you. You are all walking along towards that giant rocket. You look down at yourself and see the suit that you are wearing and you are carrying the helmet at the moment and you feel the weight of the suit and perhaps you can be surprised that the suit isn't as hot as you expected it to be for something that is so big and so heavy and surprised that you can move so easily in the suit. And you see people taking photos of you and your fellow astronauts as you walk towards the rocket and you can see the clear blue sky above you, feel the warmth of the sun, smelling the fresh air, hearing the murmuring sounds of the people, feeling a little bit in awe of the size of that rocket as you get closer to it and realising how small you appear next to it. And as you get closer to the rocket, so you and your fellow astronauts enter a lift that takes you up what looks like scaffolding up to the height of the entrance to the rocket and you let some of the other astronauts go first and then you walk out behind them and you admire the view from being so high up and you think to yourself that it is like standing at the top of the Eiffel Tower and you walk along the platform and you can hear the echoey metallic sound of each step you take and you enter the shuttle, closing the door behind you, hearing the sound of the door closing and you can feel the weight of the door as you close the door, although you can feel the door is heavy, it feels surprisingly smooth and manoeuvrable and moves with ease and you get into your seat and put your helmet on and twist it slightly to lock it in place and you can notice how you can now hear your breathing from within your helmet and notice how different the breathing sounds now breathing inside the helmet and you strap yourself in and think to yourself how awkward it is getting into the seat and strapping yourself in, when you are having to climb into the seat and lift your legs up, almost like sitting in a seat that is lying on its back.

Then you hear mission control begin to count down. They let you know everything is okay, the checks have all been done, we are safe for take-off, then they begin to count down, 10, 9, 8 and as they count down, your mind begins to focus, 7, 6, 5, 4, 3 and at three you hear a rumbling as the burners are lit, 2 and you hear a rumbling coming from the rockets, 1, 0 and on the count of zero, there is a moments pause and then suddenly what feels like an earthquake around you, a rumbling, tumbling earthquake, if there were things that could rattle you know they would. And you feel like you are lifting and you don't quite recognise it as lifting and you can't see anything outside other than a little bit of blue sky and so you can't notice that you are lifting and then after a second or two suddenly you start to feel really heavy and find yourself pushed back in your seat and after five seconds you feel like you have tripled in weight. And the rocket continues to accelerate and it quickly breaks the speed of sound and all of a sudden there is silence from outside, as you are travelling faster than the sound is able to travel from the rockets to your ears.

The acceleration continues, the sky begins to get darker and darker outside and you are aware that you must be rising up higher and higher in the earth's atmosphere. After about 15 seconds, you begin to, notice yourself becoming weightless. Suddenly the shuttle twists and turns. Out of the window you see the earth. Like a giant blue marble in space. You enjoy in awe, the view, gazing down at the earth, as the shuttle begins to circle the earth. And you unbuckle yourself and notice how you are weightless and everything just floats. And you explore the shuttle. And this isn't an ordinary shuttle, this is the latest shuttle, for a new kind of trip to space.

Part of your role in space, is to go and do a spacewalk. You have got to take a specific satellite out of the shuttle with you, just a small satellite and you have got to unfurl its solar panels, attach a few pieces to it and do all that far enough away from the shuttle, that there is no risk to the shuttle or to the satellite. And so, you leave the shuttle on your spacewalk. And you work on sorting out that satellite and you wonder what the satellite is for. You know it is to help with communication but you don't know in what context. And it is hard work to work on the satellite, but you enjoy it because you are out in space. While you are working on the satellite, a part of your mind is wondering about how in space there is no up nor down, no left, nor right, no backwards or forwards, there just is. You are aware that to you, you feel like you are stationary, sorting out a satellite, you can notice that the earth is moving beneath you, but you don't feel like you are moving. And yet you are aware that you are actually travelling around the earth at thousands of miles per hour. And you are aware that you are ageing at a different speed to your family back on earth. And so you start to ponder what reality is, if you can be travelling at thousands of miles per hour and feel like you are stationary and if you can be ageing slower than family on earth.

Once you have sorted the satellite out, you let go of it, having pressed in some codes and it autocorrects, gets itself to the correct orbit and you head back to the shuttle. Then the shuttle has a few days of orbiting the earth, where you do a few science experiments and relax, you take photos of the night sky, you take photos of the earth, you get a new perspective on things from up here, you learn and grow and after a few days in space, it is time for you to return back to earth. As you buckle back into the shuttle, the trajectory of the shuttle is changed. You begin to make the journey back down into the earth's atmosphere and as you journey back down into the earth's atmosphere, so you journey deeper asleep. You feel so relaxed journeying down into the earth's atmosphere, aware of how well built the shuttle is, how successful the shuttle is landing. Being able to enjoy the journey back down, noticing how the blackness of space starts to change to a blue of the atmosphere, passing through layers of cloud, before heading for a giant runway, landing on that runway, firing parachutes out the back of the shuttle to decelerate the shuttle and being welcomed home, almost like a hero's welcome, because, although space flight is now more common, it is still not something everyone does all the time. And you can look forward to your next space flight, to the next time you get called upon to repair a satellite, to take a satellite into space. And you can drift comfortably asleep now.

CHAPTER 16

Deep Sleep Hypnosis Session 1

Welcome.

This is going to be a thirty-minute guided hypnosis session to help you drift off into a deep and relaxing sleep. The most important thing to do while listening to this session is to keep an open mind. You must go with the flow, listen to my voice, and remember to breathe.

Remember, it is not always possible to enter a light hypnotic state on the first try, but we are going to try as I guide you gently and smoothly into this state so you can fall asleep. Please bear in mind that you are not going to enter any sort of deep catatonic state. Nothing is going to be physically altered within the realm of your mind. The process of hypnosis and this guided meditation is extremely safe, and you are in control of it.

Now, I want you to get comfortable. Because you are trying to achieve a deep sleep, you should be lying down, your head resting on your most comfortable pillow and you are warmed by your softest blanket. Lie back and let your shoulders go slack, relaxing against the cushion of your bed. Gently close your eyes and release all the tension from your muscles. Release the tension in your arms, then your legs. Let go of the tension in your chest and in your back. All of the muscles in your body begin to feel looser and looser and your body is feeling light.

Focus your attention on your toes. Softly wiggle all ten toes once, and then again. Feel the energy released from your movement and the stillness that follows. Your toes are now ready for sleep.

Next, tighten the muscles in your calves and hold for one, two, three seconds. Now release the muscles. Tighten them again for one, two, three seconds. Now release. The excess energy that keeps you up at night has been expelled from your calves. Your calves are now ready for sleep.

Next, squeeze your thigh muscles and hold for one, two, three seconds. Now release. The tension that was once stored there has been released. Your thighs are now ready for sleep. Feel the lightness that has cloaked your legs. Your legs feel weightless as if they could float up to the ceiling.

Focus your attention on your buttocks. Tighten your muscles in buttocks for one, two, three seconds. Now release the muscles. The tightness in your buttocks and lower back has been relieved. Your buttocks and lower back are now ready for sleep.

Focus your attention on your abdomen. Squeeze your abdominal muscles for one, two, three seconds. Now release. The anxiety that has been stored up and deterring sleep has been released. Your abdomen is now ready for sleep.

Concentrate on your chest. Tighten the muscles in your chest for one, two, three seconds. Now release. The sadness that has been weighing on you and preventing your mind from resting has been expelled. Your chest is now ready for sleep.

Direct your attention now to your shoulders. Tighten the muscles in your shoulder for one, two, three seconds. Now release. The stress that has been building in the deep tissue of your shoulders has now been dissolved. Your shoulders are now ready for sleep.

Focus your attention on your neck. Gently tighten the muscles and hold for one, two, three seconds. Now release. Gently tighten the muscles in your jaw and hold for one, two, three seconds. Now release. Gently tighten the muscles in your mouth and hold for one, two, three seconds. Now release. Gently squeeze your eyelids tighter for one, two, three seconds. Now release. The tension that was held in your face has now been released.

The entirety of your body has been washed with serenity as you expel the negative energy from your muscles. Now that your body is relaxed, your mind can now relax in preparation for deep slumber. Realize how free it feels to let go of all built up tension. In this moment nothing else matters. You are free. You are relaxed. You are weightless.

There is nowhere for you to be and you have everything you need. You are here, in this moment, permitting the calming sensation to course through your body. Your thoughts drift away. You don’t try to follow or catch them. With each breath you take, you are feeling more and more serene. Breathe in, welcoming peace and harmony to your soul. Breathe out, exhaling all the negative energy and releasing your control. Realize how good it feels to be so relaxed.

Focus on being as relaxed as you can be at this moment. Allow your mind to settle down a little, to quiet, to be still. Instead, focus more on your body. How does it feel lying in your bed? Examine the coziness you feel beneath your sheets. Feel how smooth your sheets are and gentle weight of your blanket on top of you. Relax in the embrace of the softest bed in the world. You are content in every way.

Imagine that on the other side of the room is an open fire crackling. The orange and yellow flames emanate a sensation of calmness as its soft light can be seen upon your walls and ceiling. You feel the warmth of this sensation. You watch closely as the flames flicker and dance upon the logs. The sound of the crackling fire reminds you that you are safe in this space. In this bed you are warm, cozy, and protected.

Scan your body for tension. Find where you still hold stress in your body. Examine your shoulders, your neck, your temples, and your back. Find the stress that is hiding and release it. Allow your body to feel relieved, relaxed, at peace.

Examine the aroma of the fire as it fills the room. The fragrance is deep and musky. It reminds you of good memories with the ones who love you. These memories remind you that your life is beautiful. Place both hands on your stomach, one below your ribs and one above your belly button. Take a deep breath in through your nose, inhale those good memories. Let the air fill your belly and your hands rise on top of your abdomen. Then, through your nose, exhale all of the negativity you have collected. The worries that you harbor are no longer welcome here.

Breathe in the relaxing scent of the fireplace, fill up your stomach like it is a balloon. Let your hands move as your inhale. Then exhale any remaining tension. You now feel loose and at ease. There is a calmness that envelopes your body as you breathe. As you feel more relaxed, you hear only the fire in this quiet space. The quietness of the room also quiets your mind and you welcome rest and relaxation.

As you lay, keep breathing and reveling in this blissful setting: you're tucked inside your cozy bed with a fire to keep you warm.

Focus on this serene moment and give yourself permission to enjoy it. Remember that you are in control. Many times, your mind is overthinking, overanalyzing, and too critical. In this moment, it is you who is in control and you will exhale those negative thoughts. As you exhale, you regain your balance and you feel content. Your body feels looser, lighter, and a weight is lifted off your chest.

Your body is light and warm as you listen to my voice. Let me guide you as you drift off. I'm going to count now and you will listen. Let my voice lull you. You are safe and relaxed and warm.

Ten... Your body is entirely loose and relaxed.

Nine... You are in a peaceful, calm, and safe environment.

Eight... You can feel the warmth and love of those who care about you, enveloping your senses.

Seven... The sound of the burning fire, the crackling of wood lulls you further into an even deeper state of relaxation.

Six... You inhale all of the good in the world with each breath you take.

Five... You exhale all the bad, expelling all of your stress and anxiety with each breath out.

Four... You feel your body getting lighter until you are almost like a feather in the breeze.

Three... You feel your mind becoming heavier and brimming with warmth and love.

Two... Accept the peace that has engulfed you, understand that it is good. Let it send you off ever deeper into the feeling of relaxation.

One... You feel yourself drifting all the way down, as deep as you can go, nearer to the bottom, towards warmth and sleep.

You are safe and you are relaxed. Allow yourself to feel safe and relaxed in this space.

Imagine that you are a leaf on a tree. You are connected to a giant colony of other leaves attached to a branch. That branch is attached to a trunk. You are a part of a busy, ever rustling tree. However, you want to be still. You need to rest. You need to separate yourself from the busyness of your world. You decide that you will depart your branch and you begin to float. Slowly, as if gravity has slowed your fall, you twirl and roll in the breeze. You are peacefully drifting further and further, reassured that you are safe.

Instead of the ground, you see that there is a quiet pond below your tree and soon you will touch the surface. As you float towards it, you notice its stillness. There are no ripples or disturbances. The surface is smooth and clear; it is as reflective as a mirror. As you reach the water, you greet the surface with a delicate kiss.

You send gentle, peaceful ripples from your contact. Concentric circles echo out to the edges of the pond. This energy radiates from you until the last ripple falls away. It is now you on the water, undisturbed and immersed in the tranquility of your setting. You drift on the surface of your unconsciousness. You feel the warmth of the water beneath you and surrounding you. The water is so soothing that you feel yourself getting heavier. You feel as though you could keep floating deeper and deeper beneath the surface until you fell asleep.

The relaxation that you feel now is beckoning you closer to rest, to deep sleep. Notice how relaxed you are in this very moment. Notice how soothing the sensations are in your body. Breathe in the relaxation that the water provides. Breathe out any tension you have.

I am going to count down from five. When I reach one, you are going to fully embrace the peace that has engulfed you and lose yourself in sleep. You will feel yourself slipping into a calm and serene rest.

Five... You think of the still surface of the pond, and how it provided safety for you, the leaf. The calm water is summoning your sleep.

Four... You feel the warmth of tranquility ripple from the top of your scalp and down your neck. It glides through your shoulders, radiates through your chest and stomach, and finally glazes over your legs. You are encompassed by this sensation.

Three... You feel your body become heavy and you softly sink in a little deeper to your consciousness. You are safe and protected.

Two... You feel yourself drift away, like your leaf on the still pond. You float away, quietly into the night.

One... You are now asleep, resting and at peace.

Breathe in, Breathe out. Breathe in, Breathe out. When you wake up, you will be renewed and refreshed and ready to take on the day. You will be ready to conquer the obstacles of your life now that you have conquered sleep.

CHAPTER 17

Saving Sally

Tessa and Natasha were going out on a bicycle ride. Their favourite place to ride was along the river and down to the ocean. There was such a fantastic path running alongside the river and they always found something exciting along the way.

The girls were both 8 years old. They had lived next door to each other their entire lives. They both loved riding their bikes, reading, playing soccer, playing the piano, swimming and anything that had anything to do with animals.

Today was the first day of the holidays and they were celebrating with a ride to the beach and a picnic on their favourite rock. One of their favourite pastimes was to sit with a good book and keep an eye on all the sea creatures busy on the beach.

They had carefully planned their picnic lunch and they were busy packing it into a little cooler bag that fit perfectly in the basket on the front of Tessa's bicycle. They packed oranges and pretzels to have as a snack along the river path. They packed peanut butter and cucumber sandwiches; a tomato, feta and olive salad (and they put some salad dressing in a small little bottle), breadsticks and hummus, and a big bottle of water. They also took lots of biscuits that they had baked with Tessa's mom the day before.

They were both wearing large summer hats and they had their bathing suits underneath their summer dresses. They put some sun lotion on, packed their books and a blanket to sit on in Natasha's basket and they were off on their way.

The path snaked around their houses and crossed over the river with a rickety wooden bridge. They took a nice easy ride as the path undulated up and over little grassy mounds, backwards and forwards over the river. Soon they came to a perfect spot to stop and have their snack.

It was a very hot day and the girls were sweating. "Tasha, let's dip ourselves in the river," said Tessa. "It's the first day of summer and it is already so hot!"

"Oooooooooh, the water is going to be freezing!" whined Natasha. "I'll probably get brain freeze!"

"Don't be silly! We'll warm up quickly as soon as we start riding our bikes again" said Tessa taking her hat and her dress off and hanging them on her bicycle. She jumped into the river and had to hold her breath to stop herself from crying out from the cold. "Don't do it Tasha!" she squealed. "My blood has just frozen!"

Natasha couldn't stop laughing as Tessa jumped out of the water quicker than she had jumped in. She shivered and shuddered her way back onto her bicycle to try and warm up again. Her whole bicycle shook as she tried to continue riding down the path.

After a short ride, Natasha called out to her friend, "Oh come on Tess! It can't be THAT bad! Stop making all those noises!"

"It's not me!" shouted Tessa. "What IS it though?"

The girls brought their bikes to a skidding halt. Something was making a very strange sound. It sounded like a mix of a mew and a ha-ha-ha-ha. They looked at each with a puzzled look on their faces. "We need to investigate this," said Natasha. "Let's put our bikes to the side and see what it is. I think something needs our help."

The girls leant their bikes against a tree and slowly started walking around. The sound stopped for a little while and then it started again: mew, mew, ha-ha-ha-ha. They looked behind bushes, they looked under bushes and they walked all the way around large trees, and then in a small opening they saw what was making that sound. A seagull was struggling going round and round in circles with one wing neatly folded onto its body and the other one dragging on the ground next to it.

"Oh no!" cried Tessa as she bent over to gently speak to the seagull. "Hello my sweet baby seagull. What happened to your wing little one? Are you okay baby girl? Oh sweet, sweet Sally! What can I do to help?"

Natasha smiled a sad smile at her friend. "Sally?" she asked.

"It's definitely Sally! And something is very wrong. What are we going to do? We can't just leave her here!"

"We are absolutely not going to leave her here," said Natasha jumping into action. "We must help her. And I think I've got an idea. Our vet has got pictures of birds all over his office. I'm sure Dr Taylor can help Sally. Let's take her there right now!" She jumped up and went to fetch the blanket from her basket while Tessa continued to reassure Sally the Seagull that they were not going to hurt her and that they would help her.

When Natasha came back she gently put the blanket over Sally's head, carefully tucked her wing close to her body and wrapped her whole little body in the blanket. She then placed Sally in her basket and the girls turned their bicycles around to go back towards the vet's office.

They tried to cycle as fast and as carefully as they could so that they didn't make Sally too scared. When they finally arrived at Dr Taylor's rooms they were puffing and panting and completely out of breath. Natasha carefully took Sally out of the basket; they carried her inside and as soon as they saw Dr Taylor's assistant they began explaining in bursts of emotion what had happened.

"Slow down girls! Slow down. Follow me straight into Dr Taylor's office and you can explain everything directly to him," said the assistant.

"Natasha, Tessa," said Dr Taylor greeting them warmly. "What brings you here? What have you got there?"

"Oh Dr Taylor you have to help us!" blurted out Tessa. "We were on our way to the beach through the forest and we found Sally in a clearing. First we heard her and we could hear something was wrong. And then when we found her we saw that there was something wrong with her wing. Something was very wrong!"

“Ok, ok. Slow down sweetheart. First things first, who is Sally?” asked Dr Taylor gently.

“Sally the Seagull!” the girls blurted out together as they gently handed the precious bird to Dr Taylor. He slowly lifted the blanket off the seagull while constantly speaking in a very low tone and with a very calm voice: “There there little one, let’s see what’s happened to your wing precious birdie.”

After examining her carefully, Dr Taylor shook his head. “I’m sorry to say that this doesn’t look good girls,” he said. “Our feathered friend has broken her wing very badly. We have two options that we have to think about very carefully. The first option is that we do an operation to amputate her wing. Birds have very small hearts but she’s a strong seagull and she could survive it. If she does survive the operation, you’ll have to help her find a good place to live that’s sheltered and protected. You’ll have to help her slowly work out how to live without flying.”

The girls glanced at each other and carried on listening.

“Seagulls eat lots of different types of food and she could maybe survive without flying. There are lots of creatures on the ground that she could catch and eat. If we chose this option, I would ask that you two keep an eye on her though and bring her back to me when I need to see her.”

Dr Taylor continued slowly choosing his words carefully, “The second option would be to say goodbye to her. She cannot survive the way she is now. I would have to end it for her.”

“No Dr Taylor, absolutely NOT!” cried out Tessa while Natasha buried her head into her hands.

“Before you girls decide, I want you to know that even if we do the operation, it doesn’t mean that she will survive it. She may die on the operating table. Or she may survive the operation and only live for a short while after that,” said Dr Taylor.

“But at least we will have given her a chance to survive,” said Natasha. “We owe it to her. We cannot just give up on her. She called us to her. It’s important that we do everything we can.”

Dr Taylor smiled kindly at the girls and said, "Would you like me to leave you alone to think about it and discuss it before you decide?"

"No," said Tessa. "I completely agree with Tasha. We absolutely must do everything we can to help her. Sally asked us for help and that is exactly what we are going to try and do."

The girls each gave Sally a little kiss on her head. They were quite surprised how she had sat on the table and had been so still while they were discussing what to do. It was almost as though she knew exactly what was being said. They whispered a little prayer in her ear and left her in the loving doctor's hands. They then decided to have their picnic on the grass outside Dr Taylor's rooms while they waited for the operation to be done.

They slowly ate the little bits that they could manage while they spoke about everything that had happened. They chose to feel optimistic about the operation and started planning how they would take care of their one-winged pet. And before they knew it, Dr Taylor was walking across the grass towards them.

"I'm trying to work out who is the most blessed one here today," he said with a tear in his eye. "Is it Sally the Seagull who knew that you two girls passing by were the ones that would help her? Is it the two of you who gave your hearts so completely and saved a beautiful soul's life? Or is it me that was lucky enough to be part of this miracle?"

"SHE MADE IT!" the girls screamed out in unison. They gave Dr Taylor the biggest hug as they all laughed and cried. They thought they had had an adventurous day but they realised that their biggest adventure was only just beginning!

CHAPTER 18

The Kingdom Without A King

Long-time ago in the ancient kingdom of Agartha, they lived a king whose name was Bran the third. King Bran had two sons, Prince Heren the elder son and heir to the throne of Agartha, and Prince Korah the younger one. Both of them were valiant men who had proved their worth both on and off the battlefield. They both lived happily with their wives. Doren the wife of Prince Heren and Maureen the wife of Prince Korah. Their wives would often pray together for their husbands whenever they went out for battle.

The city of Agartha has been besieged for over two weeks and the people were beginning to starve and there was a massive uproar. King Bran had to something and he had to so really fast. He wasn't prepared to risk the lives of thousands of his soldiers and his sons. He thus suggested a one on one duel with King Nemroth who had led the siege against Agartha. King Nemroth eventually agreed to the terms laid out by King Bran and a day was set for the duel. It was agreed that whosoever won the duel had automatically won the battle for his city.

The day of reckoning came and over 30,000 soldiers surrounded the battleground waiting to strike in case anything goes wrong with the agreement. While the people of Agartha were already starving from hunger, they remained committed and dedicated to protecting their city. Agartha prior to that moment has not lost a single battle since their history. It was a record worth protecting and King Bran would do everything humanly possible to ensure he keeps this record alive.

Many men of valour had willingly volunteered to represent Agartha in the duel including General Smith who was head of the Agarthanian army. King Bran turned down all their aspirations and insisted he was the one to take on King Nemroth's fighter. The two princes of Agartha tried all means to stop their father from partaking in the duel for he was already getting weary out of old age. King Bran, as usual, was a very stubborn and persistent king who would love to lay down his life for his people anytime occasion demands such. This was one of those rare instances and he had to prove to his people yet again that he was still their servant despite being a king.

King Bran somehow managed to overpower and win King Nemroth's soldier who was a giant, but not without a deep wound on his right leg. However, King Bran did have the opportunity to kill King Nemroth's giant, but decided to spare his life, leaving King Nemroth with no choice than to honour the agreement between both kingdoms. He subsequently retrieved his armies and called off the siege. Normalcy and tranquility were once again restored to the city of Agartha. This was hugely hinged on the selfless act displayed by the king of Agartha.

For over three months, King Bran remained on the sick bed and all efforts to heal his wounded leg proved abortive. The kingdom of Agartha slowly began to weaken and King Bran just had to proclaim an heir to the throne to take over from him. His heir would be no other than Prince Heren who had shown utmost loyalty, dedication, and commitment to serving the kingdom of Agartha.

'I King Bran the third, name you Prince Heren of Agartha the king of Agartha in my stead. Arise Oh King' King Bran concluded as he made his elder son the king of Agartha. Everyone had gathered to witness the great occasion. There was wild jubilation amongst the people and they all rushed to give gifts and goodwill to their new king. It was indeed a joyful sight to behold. A few days later, King Bran was called to the great beyond and he had no choice than to answer the call.

King Heren ruled powerfully and wisely and maintained the good legacy left by his father. With the support of his younger brother, he conquered so many kingdoms and the fame of Agartha grew under his stead. While King Bran was more of a patient king, his successor, King Heren wasn't. He often went full-fledged into battles and luckily for him he succeeds in all.

As fate would have it, both the king and his younger brother's wife both got pregnant at about the same time and fortunately, they both gave birth the same day. Both the king and his younger brother were drinking and making merry that night when their wives went into the labour room. Their joy heightened when one of the maidens broke the good news of safe delivery to them. Prince Korah leapt for joy and ran out to celebrate with some of his friends. He never bothered to ask of his baby's gender, all he cared was that both his wife and his brother's wife had delivered safely. However, King Heren asked the maid the gender of both children which the maiden did and also enthusiastically told the King those present when the babies were born. The smile and joy on King Heren's face turned instantly and he was visibly filled with rage and anger. How could my brother's wife give birth to a male child while mine gave birth to a female child? he pondered. This can't be he exclaimed.

In the kingdom of Agartha, females are forbidden to rule over the kingdom. In cases were the king doesn't have a male heir to the throne, the crown falls to the next legitimate male heir who in this case was going to be his brother's child. Having spent so many years looking for a child, and heading out for numerous battles, King Heren couldn't take any chances letting her brother's child survive. He immediately conjured up a plan with General Smith to kill his own daughter and exchange her for his brother's wife's son.

Needless to say, the sheer ruthlessness of General Smith ensured the plan went according to plan and to seal the secret, the maiden who broke the news to King Heren was lured to the city walls and killed by General Smith. Her body was carefully disposed of and no one ever heard of her again. Prince Korah was so saddened following the untimely demise of his daughter as the case may be. He lost all zeal and enthusiasm to contribute towards the affairs of the kingdom. He left the castle and lived a low life with his wife afterward.

However, two years later, his wife gave birth to another child. This time a girl, but Prince Korah cared less. A child was a child to him regardless of gender. He was all joy yet again and smile was restored to his face. King Heren led his royal entourage to visit his brother on the day of the child's naming ceremony and the child was named Litica by her father. King Heren urged his brother to come back to the castle and live together with them, but he turned it down. Prince Korah said he preferred living among the common men and feeling like one of them. After much persuasion he allowed his grown-up daughter, Litica to go back to the castle to live with the King and his family.

Growing up in the castle was entirely different for Litica as compared to how she was brought up during her childhood outside the castle. Everything she needed was made readily available to her, and to Litica's life in the castle was all so boring. Save for Arnold who was her cousin or perhaps more correctly her brother, she had absolutely no one else to play with.

Arnold, on the other hand, was way too comfortable in the castle. He was brought up poorly with little or no idea on how to go about basic household chores. He would often eat, sleep and play around the castle. Litica found this boring and would often sneak out of the castle to be thought how to shoot the arrow by General Smith. She learnt how to use the sword and the arrow after so many practices and lessons from General Smith.

King Heren was becoming uneasy with the closeness of his head of the army and his brother's daughter. He feared that one day, General Smith may eventually speak up and say the truth of what happened many years ago. He plotted to eliminate the last person who was the evidence of the evil act he perpetrated. On one fateful evening, King Heren invited General Smith for dinner. Unknowingly to General Smith that King Heren had poisoned his drink. He came to visit the king for dinner as he does on rare occasions especially when the king had something troubling him.

General Smith arrived just in time as the table for dinner was set. The king had a very long chit-chat with him without discussing anything serious. Though General Smith was surprised the king didn't have anything important to discuss with him, he didn't hesitate to eat the delicious food and gulp down the drinks on the dining table.

The whole kingdom was thrown into a state of mourning and grief following the news of General Smith's untimely demise. He was greatly loved for his loyalty, charming smile and tactical prowess on the field of battle. The Agarthanian army mourned General Smith for about 21 days and some of them even quit the army. It was a time of deep contrition for everyone in the kingdom, both old and young, big and small.

Prince Korah couldn't eat for two days on hearing the sad news. He had no idea what could have killed a young valiant soldier like Smith, but whatever it was, he wished him well as he sojourned to the great beyond. Litica and Arnold did not feel any different about the death of Smith. To Litica she had lost a great companion and mentor who regularly taught her how to use the sword and arrow.

King Heren wasted no time in appointing a replacement for Smith. Practically though it was nearly impossible to replace someone as good as Smith especially on the battlefield. After scouting for a near-perfect replacement, the King chose Agadon, the brother of Obed the great seer of Agartha and made him head over the army.

King Heren went continued his dominance over the land going on to conquer even more territories and his fame increased and spread across the face of the earth, but so did his bloodthirst. He would often neglect the needs of his people and set out conquering weak and smaller kingdoms who look up to him for strength and security. King Heren went as far as going to battle with King Nemroth and his great army. Little did he know he was going to meet his waterloo. The Agarthanian was utterly defeated and brought to nothing.

King Heren was injured severely in the battle and his army was well massacred without any form of mercy. If there was a disgraceful outing, this battle was a perfect definition of it. Perhaps due to the absence of General Smith whom the soldiers loved and respected or the sheer stubbornness of King Heren who failed to heed to the counsel of Obed the great seer. The armies of Agartha fought rather timidly and were easily overpowered by their enemies. King Heren eventually came back to Agartha through an escape route with a handful of soldiers. King Heren had set out for that battle with about 20,000 soldiers, but returned with about 2,000. Such was the severity of the damage done and for the very first time since King Bran the 1st, the Agarthanian army tasted defeat.

King Heren though critically ill as a result of the wound he sustained in battle still monitored his son closely. He saw very little or no attribute of a good leader in him. he was so lackadaisical and reluctant in everything he did save for his flute which he was adept with and loved playing. This became a major cause of worry for the king as Litica, on the other hand, was everything he wanted in a successor. She was brave, hardworking, intelligent and caring. She would sometimes sneak out of the castle to assist the poor old men and women and anyone else who needed her assistant. All this she did with utmost humility.

King Heren would have loved to proclaim a new king of Agartha as he was not getting any better. The knowledge of giving the throne and handing over power to Arnold who was ideally his brother's son bothered him and gave him sleepless nights. He was confused and so reluctant to hand over power to Arnold not necessarily because he was truly his brother's child, but because to him, Arnold lacked the capacity to competence to rule the great kingdom of Agartha.

King Heren finally resolved to seek for the guidance of Obed the great seer of Agartha. King Heren tearfully told Obed all that had transpired in the past and how General Smith was killed. However, he asked for forgiveness of the Gods and the way to remedy the situation. The counsel of Obed was sought and he proffered a solution to the king. Both Litica and Arnold were to sojourn to Irkalla, the land of no return to retrieve the lost cup of life and whoever came back alive with it would be crowned king.

Litica and Arnold were equipped with everything they needed. While Litica was armed with her sword, arrow, and armour, Arnold took only his flute. Left for him there was absolutely no need of going to the land of no return when the people do not expect them to return. It just didn't make sense to him. While he saw it either as a mere waste of time or a death sentence, Litica saw it as an adventure and an opportunity to showcase the skills which she had learnt over the years from General Smith and her father.

Litica and Arnold were accompanied by a host of soldiers and other concerned persons until they got to the shore of the river Tibbeth. From there both Litica and Arnold were expected to continue their sojourn all alone. Litica who had been around the poor old men and women had heard several stories about Irkalla and it was time for her to witness how true the legends were. On the shore of the river was an old rickety looking boat with a very old fiery man on it. It was the only means to get to the entrance of Irkalla and the old man demanded one coin each from both of them.

Litica having heard stories about the journey to Irkalla came along with just two coins. One for the ferryman when she was going and the other when she was coming back. Arnold had no coins with him and both of them had to continue the journey. Litica having very little or no option decided to have compassion on Arnold and gave the ferryman both coins in her possession.

The ferryman took the coins and crossed them over to the other side of the river to Irkalla. On stepping down from the boat, the old looking ferryman who had been speaking so faintly spoke and sounded exactly like General Smith and all Litica could remember was 'what is lost may never be lost' don't forget that in your quest for the cup of life.' Litica and Arnold jolted up to find themselves in a maze with no idea how they got there nor how they were going to leave.

Well, maybe this is Irkalla, the land of no return said, Arnold. I think I like it here for we aren't going back anyway. Before he could complete his statement, Litica had already embarked on her adventure, seeking for the cup of life. They both ran around and searched frantically around the maze for the cup of life. They were sometimes attacked by huge creatures that were defeated by Litica.

Litica and Arnold had searched for the cup of life for over five days with very little progress made. They would often get back to the exact spot they started on the maze each time they set out for the quest. On the sixth day of their quest, Arnold became so weak and weary and opted to quit the quest and rather play his flute instead. He played his flute with melodious songs over and over and over again. Little did he know he was summoning Eunice the goddess of music and dance who had been trapped forever in the land of no return.

A beautiful lady clads in a glowing white apparel appeared right in front of Arnold dancing. Arnold overlooked the presence of this strange creature and focused on playing his flute. He was already in another world; the goddess of music has perhaps possessed him to play continual melodious songs for her. The goddess's fun was caught short as Litica aimed two arrows in quick succession to the strange creature whom she feared was about to attack Arnold. To Litica's disbelief, she failed to kill this creature, unlike others. She became really terrified and ran off and before she could summon enough courage to face the strange creature again, it had already disappeared. What shocked most was that Arnold was awake, hale and hearty without as much as a scratch.

Before Eunice left, however, the goddess gave him the chance to make two wishes. Firstly, he requested that the goddess guide them in getting the cup of life. However, he reserved the second wish for subsequent use. The goddess had handed over to him a small round object which would serve as a pointer to them in the direction they would go. After much thorough search, the pointer finally led them to the cup of life located right at the middle of four fierce-looking lions apparently guiding the cup. Now the cup has been seen, how do they get it out of the place alive was a big question which perturbed them.

Litica somehow managed to overpower and kill all four lions and grabbed the cup of life. Just as she did, the grounds quaked and there was turbulence all over the place. Arnold was under intense pressure from Litica to use his last wish to get them out of the place alive. However, he had earlier promised to use one of his wish to set Eunice free. He was stuck between keeping his word and fighting for his own safety. Though he might not return, he wished that Eunice be released from the trap of the land of no return. Immediately Eunice was free and Irkalla was filled with melodious songs. The turbulence subsided and Litica was shocked. Perhaps, Arnold took the right decision for once in his life. They both headed back to the entrance of the maze which was very difficult to locate, but for the guidance of the pointer.

On getting to the entrance, they were faced with another challenge. They had used both coins that were with them to come, going back thus became a near-impossible task. Again, Eunice came to their rescue and made them an offer. If she would provide two coins for them to sail back, then they would have to use the cup of life to transform her fully back to human form. After extended deliberations between Litica and Arnold, they both agreed to her request. They were given two coins for the ferryman and Litica, in turn, used the cup of life to transform her back to her normal self.

The goddess turned out to be a very beautiful maiden and little did Litica know that the cup of life could only be used once before it loses its possess until retrieved again from Irkalla. Both Litica, Arnold and the maiden set sail after giving the ferryman two coins. They were astonished why the ferryman didn't collect a coin from the maiden. This wasn't much of their concern though, they just had to get back home safely.

The people of Agartha couldn't contain their joy as they saw Litica and Arnold arrive. They weren't sure who the last person among them was though. Litica and Arnold along with the damsel were led to the castle amidst rejoicing and dancing. The songs they heard and danced to were so melodious, such that has never been singing in the kingdom. On stepping into the castle chambers, King Heren fell down on his knees and pleaded profusely for forgiveness. His brother, Prince Korah and all-around had no idea why he was doing this except Obed who just stools smiling.

King Heren explained to everyone the wicked misdeed he had done to his brother and his wife, how he had killed the maiden who came to share the news through General Smith and how he had also killed General Smith to safeguard his secret. To the utter consternation of the already teeming crowd, the damsel who stood before him with Litica and Arnold was the same maiden he had killed many years ago. The cup of life was useless to him as he could no longer use it to save himself. He pleaded that his brother and the people of Agartha forgive him.

Some persons picked up stones to stone King Heren to death, but Prince Korah intervened urging the people of Agartha to forgive and forget. With tears in his eyes, he pitifully forgave his brother. King Heren thus made his last proclamation as king before he gave up the ghost. He overruled the law that stated only males are allowed to inherit the throne of Agartha and replaced with the Council of Leaders which would consist of everyone from the royal family and one representative from each constituent clan of Agartha kingdom. Thus he proclaimed and he lived no more. From that day henceforth, the great kingdom of Agartha never had a king till this day, but a Council of Leaders who governed the affairs of the kingdom.

CHAPTER 19

THE SCULPTURE INSIGHT

Steps for increasing effectiveness of the story:

1. What do you want to achieve from reading this?
2. Think about one thing you have achieved today.
3. Say to yourself "When I read this story then..."

Alternative introduction:

"As I read this and begin to drift comfortably asleep, I don't know whether I will find myself drifting asleep more to the sound of my voice or the words I read, or perhaps to the spaces between the words. And as I drift comfortably asleep I'll just read this story to myself."

So as you listen to me and you begin to comfortably fall asleep, I don't know whether you will fall asleep quicker with the sound of my voice, or with the words that I use, or perhaps with the spaces between my words and as you begin to comfortably fall asleep I'm just going to tell you a story in the background and it is a story about a man who is sitting on a beach, it is a nice warm sunny day and the beach is quite quiet and he has come here to sit down and relax. And while he is sitting on the beach he is reading a book and as he is reading so his attention is being drawn into that book, drawn into the story and in the background he is aware that there is the sound of the waves lashing on the shore, aware of the sounds of birds in the sky, he is aware of distant sounds around him, he can feel the warmth of the sun on his face, he can feel what the ground feels like beneath him where he is sitting and yet his attention is drawn into the book.

And while he is reading the book, he finds that it is almost like the story jumps off the page and starts to form in his mind. As if, he starts off reading and hearing the words recited in his own voice in his mind and then gradually that reciting voice fades away to almost experiencing the story on the page and the story that he is reading is about someone out on a boat and they are heading to an island and the boat is bobbing up and down on the water and chugging through the water and it is a warm sunny day, while this boat is chugging through the water. There is blue sky, perhaps some wispy clouds, but it is a warm sunny day and as that boat continues, so the man on the boat notices the island coming into view in the distance. And continues on that boat towards that island and the boat continues to move with the waves, as well as moving through the waves.

On arrival near the island there is nowhere to dock the boat. So, the man drops anchor a little way from the island, lowers down a rigid inflatable boat off of the back of his boat into the water, climbs aboard that boat and powers towards the shore. This smaller boat, jumps and bounces on the waves as it nears the shore. The man cuts the engine and glides the boat up onto the beach. Here on the island he can hear the sounds of tropical birds, the way the water laps onto the sand, the sound of the sand beneath his feet. And he starts exploring the island.

He is here to discover something and as he explores the island, he finds a beachball that appears to have been washed up here. And almost instinctively he picks up the beachball, just to carry that beachball and to play with that beachball in his hands, he doesn't know why, it just seems to be an instinctive thing, he just saw it and picked it up and walked along tossing it gently into the air, spinning it slightly in the air, noticing the vivid, bold colours on that beachball as he throws it, catches it and spins it while he is exploring the island.

He cuts into the trees, works his way through the trees and as the trees get denser he has to put down the beachball to continue, so that he can push through those trees. And after a while he finds himself on the far side of this island, on a different beach. And on this side of the island he notices that the water is far rougher, the waves are far higher, he can see dark clouds out to sea and the occasional flash of lightning on the horizon, although it is too far to hear any rumbles of thunder. And he starts exploring this side of the island, starts exploring this beach. He doesn't know exactly what he is looking for but he knows he will recognise it when he finds it. And after some time exploring, he sees what looks like part of a chest poking out from the sand and he goes over and with his hands he digs around the chest until he can pull the chest out of the sand and onto the beach.

He breaks the lock open and opens the chest. Inside the chest he finds a book. While sat down next to the chest he starts flicking through the pages of that book, starts reading the pages of the book and looking at the images in that book. And realises that it is teaching him some kind of knowledge, something he has to do. And that it is going to take a long time to do it. He realises that this column of stone which is next to where he found the chest, that is just off the tree line, is there for a reason. He reads that he needs to carve a specific sculpture if he is to get what it is that he seeks. He reads in the book what that sculpture is supposed to look like, what carving he is supposed to do. In the chest, he sees that there is a hammer and chisel. He takes the hammer and chisel and starts chipping away at that stone, chipping away carefully in small amounts at a time, chipping away what isn't necessary, with the idea that it will leave just that which is necessary and he chips away and he chips away, as the day wears on and the sun starts to set.

He then sets up a camp on the beach for the night, lights a fire and has something to eat, falls asleep in a makeshift tent to the sounds of the water on the shore and the sight of millions of stars in the sky. The next morning after having something to eat he carries on chipping away at that stone, chipping away, carving and removing what isn't necessary, to leave what is essential. He continues to chip and carve away and by the middle of the day he begins to notice what is forming. He notices that it is starting to look like a person. He carries on chipping away and chipping away for the rest of the day and then settles down again for the night, before carrying on again the next morning. And he does this for a number of days and nights, chipping away at the sculpture, removing what isn't necessary and leaving that which is essential.

After a number of days of chipping away, he finally finishes the sculpture and sees that it looks like a person facing into the woods. But, he doesn't seem to have got what it is that he came here for. So, he doesn't fully understand. He has invested a lot of time and energy into chipping away at this sculpture and he sits down on the beach wondering what he is supposed to have learned, wondering what all of this means. He has removed all of that stone and yet this sculpture is just a sculpture of a person, it hasn't taught him anything. He has something to eat and he falls asleep that night wondering what this could all mean and he tries to let his brain process that, let his brain work on what this could all mean. He processes the last few days, processes the effort he has taken, all the information he has read. He was somehow supposed to gain knowledge from this, something that enriches your life, but he hasn't seen any treasures and he can't figure out the clue.

During his dream, he starts to have unusual thoughts, thoughts of being too warm and taking off some layers, of being too cold and putting new layers on. Thoughts of getting to know a best friend, or a loved one. By the morning, he awoke having an idea about what it is he was supposed to have learned from carving this sculpture and from chipping away all that material and leaving only that which is necessary for the sculpture. He realises that this whole journey wasn't about gaining some kind of financial incentive, it was about enriching the inner life and learning about yourself and gaining a deep knowledge about yourself, about who you are, who you want to be, how you are and how you want to be and how to get from who you are and how you are, to who you want to be and how. He realised that was what working on this sculpture had taught him. That was the insight he was supposed to gain.

As he looked at the sculpture having gained that insight, just like a snowman the sculpture seemed to melt into nothing. Almost like it was built out of sand and the sand had just collapsed to the ground merging in with the rest of the sand. He placed the book back in the chest and he reburied the chest and prepared for a journey back home. He cut back through the trees, all the way back to the beach he arrived on. Pushed his boat into the water, started the motor, travelled back to his boat, got on his boat, raised his small boat, lifted the anchor and set off homeward. And as the story ended the man closed the book aware that he had learned something about himself from this story that he had decided to read.

And while he mindfully processed that story he stood up from the beach, walked down to the shore, could feel the way the sand went from dry and grainy to damp and stodgy where his feet would sink slightly into the sand with each step. He could see the area of dryness spread from under his foot each time he placed his foot down as it compressed the sand and pushed the water out of the way. And he noticed with each step that as he raised his foot that water rushed back in again making that sand damp again. And he walked to the water's edge and he walked a little way into the water and he could feel that the sea water was warm and he could feel the movement of the water around his ankles and his feet, the way it pulled the sand in and out that he could feel through his toes, he took a few deep breaths of sea air and could feel the warmth of the sun on his face as he enjoyed and processed the insights he had gained from reading that story and allowing himself to become absorbed in that story. He processed those insights as he just listened to the natural world around him and learned about who he is and how he is in this world, what his purpose is. Those parts of him he likes and those parts of him he would like to change and shift and who he would like to be and he learned from that sculpture.

After spending some time allowing all that to integrate, he then started travelling home, still thinking about how he is integrating all of this new learning. On arrival home, he had something to eat, he relaxed for a while, before going up to bed, closing his eyes and drifting deeply and comfortably asleep. And as he drifted comfortably asleep he began to dream about being on that island, about running his hands around the sculpture, feeling the handy work that was done, feeling a connection with that work, admiring that sculpture, learning from that sculpture, feeling the smoothness of the stone to the backdrop of a distant storm as the waves lashed on the shore and he felt himself drawn deeper and deeper into this healing dream as he drifted and floated deeper and deeper asleep, internalising and understanding this in a whole new level previously unknown, learning on an instinctive level, until his dream began to fade and he began to just drift even deeper and comfortably asleep.

CHAPTER 20

Affirmations

10 Calming Bedtime Affirmations

1. I discharge today.

I let go of dread, stress, outrage, and fault. I discharge nerves and stress. I discharge the greatness of today and the weight on my shoulders. I let go of negative contemplations, and keep the upbeat ones. In my rest will I discover the opportunity to know satisfaction and harmony once more.

2. I excuse everything.

What has happened has been in this way, and there is no other way I could have or ought to have left it alone. Thus, I let it go and I let life be all things considered. I pardon the individuals, I excuse the circumstance, and I excuse myself. I believe life and I am sheltered.

3. I have authorization to nod off.

I give myself authorization to close my eyes today, and alert revived tomorrow. I am permitted to float into a decent night's rest. My body, psyche, and soul are deserving of their rest.

What I've done today is sufficient. I am and have enough, and now I permit myself an opportunity to rest.

4. I presently enter a position of profound and serene rest.

My room is a position of harmony and unwinding. At the point when I go into this room, and creep into bed around evening time, the present considerations normally start to mollify. My weight helps and rest is coming.

5. I am appreciative.

I am appreciative for this life. I am thankful for the individuals who have been my instructors. I am appreciative for the exercises life has brought. I am thankful for adoration that I get, give, and offer. I am appreciative for the light of day. I am thankful for the dimness of night, in which I will rest calmly today around evening time.

6. I grasp my fantasies.

As the night gets dull, my stresses blur. I rest calmly realizing I have done everything I could accomplish for now. I grasp my fantasies, for tomorrow will accompany another light and new quality.

I nod off with my fantasies near my heart, and everything is great.

7. May my rest be serene.

May my rest be serene. May my fantasies be loaded up with adoration. May my spirit stir to the unending conceivable outcomes for bliss in my life.

8. I welcome the characteristics of good rest.

I invite harmony into my home. I welcome light into my heart. Love, bliss, and solace reside in my spirit. My soul is content and my psyche is still. I become serene, loose. With appreciation, I respect a decent night's rest.

9. I pick harmony.

I pick harmony. I close my eyes and decide to see again with new eyes, past what my physical eyes can see. Harmony is my need. Harmony starts with me, and there is harmony in my spirit.

"Nothing can upset the quiet tranquility of my spirit." – Jiddu Krishnamurti

10. I am in amicability with the universe.

I coordinate my pulse with the beat of the universe. I am in amicability with the night and the rest that will accompany it.

There is no partition now, just a single heartbeat that thumps gradually, calmly.

CONCLUSION

Now that you have read through and practiced all the different styles of these self-guided meditations, you may be wondering what components will work the best for you depending on your needs. It will do you well to try all the different breathing patterns and visualizations to discover if something works better. Through practice and self-exploration, it is certain you will find what exactly works the best for you.

If you are having a lighter night of restlessness and need to ease down just a little to fall asleep, the meditations near the beginning of the book will work well for you. Follow the three components that make up a meditation. Begin by observing everything, your breathing your body, and what is happening in the mind. Then relax the body and find an even tone of breathing. Finally finding the stillness needed for deep rest and focusing the mind on your breath and maybe a short mantra. On nights where the weight of sleeplessness is a little lighter, you do not necessarily need to do a long drawn out visualization. A simple practice with a heavy emphasis on your breathing will probably do the trick just fine.

Help and emotional support

The same way you need to support your body throughout the process of recovery, your mind and feelings also need care and love. Being self-sufficient is a virtue, but going through depression alone, without the support of friends and family is unnecessarily burdening. Overcoming the desire to appear strong and independent might feel uncomfortable. Perhaps, you don't like to rely on others for help. But, breaking the barrier between you and your social environment is best done through the acceptance of help and care. Your support system, which may include friends and family, can lift a lot of weight off your shoulders and give you the necessary love and acceptance you need. Here's what your friends and family can help you with to support your recovery:

Household chores

Household chores tend to feel overwhelming when you're suffering from depression. If there are friends and family members willing and able to ease the load, accept all the help you can get. Fight the desire to try to do everything on your own, as it is completely unnecessary and goes against your recovery. Instead, ask for those around who are able and willing to help with cleaning, laundry, shopping, and other chores. Aside from physical help, you will have more company and you'll spend less time alone.

Paperwork

Paying bills and other paperwork may be too much to fit into your schedule, causing more anxiety and tension. Have someone take over this duty until you feel calmer and more collected. Having another task off your plate will leave you with more time for rest, relaxation, and other enjoyable activities that are beneficial to your recovery.

Financial aid

It's very likely that your symptoms have taken a toll on work and finances. If so, accept all the financial help that you can get. If you feel like you're struggling to keep up with utility bills, rent, and loans, don't hesitate to ask for help. Trying to handle all the problems on your own is likely to lead to unnecessary debt. Any sort of illness will reduce your work capacities, and the effect on finances is inevitable. If there's anyone who can provide financial aid, don't think twice about accepting it.

Socializing and outdoor activities

Getting as much fresh air as possible is beneficial for both physical and mental health, as well as connecting and socializing. Isolation is common for those who suffer from depression, and you should work to overcome the urge to be alone, even if most of the time, you want to be alone. However, schedule social activities and follow through with them regardless of whether or not you feel motivated to do so. Being more socially active is likely to be a part of your recovery plan, as well as one of the activities you can practice with behavioral activation.

Conversation and understanding

Opening up about the dark thoughts and feelings may seem difficult, but it will help you get the support you need. It's very likely that the problems will sound less dramatic than envisioned in your mind once you simply talk about them. The exaggerated thinking typical to depression is causing you to magnify everything from difficulties to feelings, fears, and doubts. Talking will help overcome many things that are bothering you, and bonding and receiving encouragement will enforce the positive beliefs you're looking to create.

Encouragement and motivation

Aside from having someone to keep you company, you need to surround yourself with people who are willing to motivate you and lift your spirits. Those should be the people you feel comfortable talking to at any time, and on any topic, because they are always willing to support. Your therapist will be among those who are supportive but make sure to open up to as many people as you trust. You'll benefit from hearing others' positive thoughts about yourself.

Compassion

Last, but not least, you need the support of those around you who are truly compassionate and willing to be accepting of your feelings. Understanding the nature of depression is not everyone's talent. The lack of compassion could worsen your desire to isolate yourself. Avoid people who are critical or are forcing you to 'cheer up' and instead look for the company of those who are able to understand your experience.

The of this book introduced you with valuable knowledge of the causes of depression and anxiety, as well as strategies to cope. The last of this book showed you what is necessary for you to do to support your own recovery. Opening up and receiving help is one of the most difficult barriers to cross with depression. The harder it is for you to ask for help, the more important it is to do it. Both subconsciously and continuously, you are working to give yourself permission to be imperfect, depend and rely on others, and receive love. Practicing connection and receiving help won't only temporarily ease your load, but help reprogram your mind in the long run.

Transitioning from Meditation to Life Scenarios

EC and the SUN meditation models are not just another fashionable hobby, but a way to survive, a way of the most painless transition to a new stage of development, and now it is vital for everyone and every day. This is a lifebuoy thrown by the light forces into the murky whirlpool of our lives and only one who is struggling for life-saving appliances, and not one who chases after a ghostly fish in muddy water will be saved. You should spare a few minutes for this simple and quite enjoyable action, because these minutes will immediately turn into hours of good mood and an enormous capacity for work, luck, and efficiency, and ultimately help to overcome unhealthy issues such as sleep anxiety, insomnia, depression, and many other life problems.

The main thing is not to know but to be able to. For example, you can read hundreds of books about how great a process heals and cleanses, but if at the same time a person has never been at this point, then all his theoretical knowledge is worthless. You can even write another book yourself on the basis of this theoretical knowledge, even with further books, research, and reasoning. But at the same time, even the most illiterate performer is much happier than such a book "attendant."

The same is true with the use of these techniques. It is important not only to learn about their existence and benefits but to be able to use them in your personal practice, in your life, in solving your life problems. Perhaps not immediately, but over time you will understand their sweet taste. The taste of cycling cannot be understood immediately, sitting on a bicycle for the first time. Time will pass, and your efforts will pay off. The acquired experience, knowledge and skills will remain for your whole subsequent life. The more often you use this meditative “magic,” the deeper you will reveal and use its versatility and power, grandeur and beauty, and the more pleasure you will experience from it.

All of these innumerable divine qualities, universality and power, harmony and beauty, and much more - every day will more and more clearly manifest in you, in your actions, thoughts, behavior, appearance, and literally everything that concerns you. Many of your life "unsolvable" problems before will suddenly begin to be resolved and sometimes even without much effort, as if by themselves. One day you will notice that many of your old sores suddenly disappeared somewhere. Then, you will notice that your touch, your look, and your very presence have a beneficial effect and even heal, if not all, then many others. Then you will find that your word, your desire, thought is being fulfilled, materializing as if by itself.

You may not know all the mechanisms of these miracles, but they will happen to you and around you more and more often. The main thing is that you will be able to create them almost effortlessly, sometimes even by accident, in passing! The Power of Love is the greatest power in the Universe! EC and SUN just teach her to awaken and be used. Every day your Rays of Love will be brighter and stronger. Every day, the Space of Love around you will be wider and more stable. Every day around you, and therefore in you, there will be more and more peace and joy, happiness and health!

SUN Meditation Text

The sun is clear, come out from behind the clouds,

light us, light our thorny path!

The sun is clear, come out from behind the clouds,

light us, light our thorny path!

And the sun is shining. He does not care:

neither wind, nor storm, nor lightning, nor thunder.

And the sun shines in the sky above

It brings joy to you and me.

And the sun shines beyond the clouds

not knowing, not knowing either captivity or fetters.

And the sun shines in the blue of heaven

and gives inspiration to you and me.

And the sun shining, bestow warmth,

It does not choose who is good and who is evil.

And the sun shining, bestow warmth,

It does not choose who is a coward and who is a hero.

And the sun shines with sacred beauty

behind clouds of dust, behind dirty vanity.

And the sun shines in everyone's chest,

how bright It is, just look!

The sun is clear, come out from behind the clouds,

light us, light our thorny path!

The sun is clear, come out from behind the clouds,

only Your Sacred Ray will save us today!

And the sun shines in peace of mind,

a melody of prayer will remind oneself.

And the sun is shining, shining and burning:

and all that is good in us, it creates!

The sun is clear, come out from behind the clouds,

light us, light our thorny path!

The sun is clear, come out from behind the clouds,

only your Sacred Ray will save us today!

The efficiency of this text depends on the person himself, and over time, this power grows. For beginners, the power of the rays is usually weak. They are still clearing their bio-field. For strong, pure-hearted people, rays can reach anywhere on the planet.

Of course, significant results here are possible only with a fairly massive application of this technique. The strength of the global impact of EC and the SUN increases significantly with:

a) an increase in the number of people using EC and the SUN;

b) increasing the frequency, regularity, and diligence of the use of EC and the SUN;

c) the synchronism (simultaneity) of the use of EC and the SUN at once by many people.

After half an hour after reading this technique or after its live demonstration, any person is already quite familiar with the EC system and can apply and use it himself. EC has the ability of self-learning because when it is used, a person receives bright energies, and with them, bright information, each time individual, unique, and necessary for this particular person. And thus, after a week of regular use, each person automatically becomes a master, which means that he can well teach it to use other people.

Of course, complete knowledge of the true capabilities of meditation cannot be achieved (and all of them cannot be achieved at all, because they are unlimited as the Universe), but in practice, these unlimited potential possibilities are limited only by the faith and diligence of each individual person. A single reading of EC can give a person more energy-knowledge than reading hundreds of books. With regular use of EC, its strength and effectiveness are steadily growing, because the rays from a person come more and more bright, stronger, and denser every day.

All surrounding people and living beings begin to feel it. And thus, even a person who does not know how to read and write can, without any additional efforts, heal diseases (his own and those around him) that did not succumb to even the best medical luminaries and academics. But this is still a child's game compared to the parallel impact of EC on global planetary processes, such as weather correction, natural disasters, crime, war, etc.

Well, less of that. It starts with you. Remember, do not try to cry at full strength, because then you quickly get tired and exhale. And do not whisper, for then meditation will be ineffective. When performed correctly, OM singing should be pleasant and somewhat reminiscent of artful massage. With too weak massage effects, muscles and skin do not receive sufficient stimulation, and such massage is ineffective. And with too strong, rough massage effects, you can damage the skin and muscles. Therefore, here we must adhere to the golden mean.

Sleep Anxiety

Thank you for picking up this book, and hopefully, you will utilize all these tools to help your insomnia. It is only a matter of time before you are sleeping soundly through the night again. I wish you the best on your journey to better nights and complete rest. May your energy be restored, and your mind be able to rest and recover down when needed. This book is entirely for you and achieving the best nights of sleep in your life.

CPSIA information can be obtained
at www.ICGtesting.com
Printed in the USA
LVHW021746150722
723616LV00018B/1453

9 781803 305387